Psychiatry
in the Nursing Home
Second Edition

Psychiatry in the Nursing Home
Second Edition

D. Peter Birkett, MD

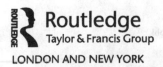

Routledge
Taylor & Francis Group

LONDON AND NEW YORK

First published 2001 by The Haworth Press

2 Park Square, Milton Park, Abingdon, Oxfordshire OX14 4RN
605 Third Avenue, New York, NY 10017

Routledge is an imprint of the Taylor & Francis Group, an informa business

First issued in paperback 2020

Copyright © 2001 Taylor & Francis

Notice:
Product or corporate names may be trademarks or registered trademarks, and are used only for identification and explanation without intent to infringe.

Cover design by Jennifer M. Gaska.

Library of Congress Cataloging-in-Publication Data

Birkett, D. Peter.
    Psychiatry in the nursing home / D. Peter Birkett.—2nd ed.
      p. ; cm.
    Includes bibliographical references and index.
    ISBN 0-7890-1214-6 (hard : alk. paper) — ISBN 0-7890-1219-7 (soft : alk. paper)
    1. Nursing home patients—Mental health. 2. Geriatric psychiatry. 3. Nursing homes. I. Title.
    [DNLM: 1. United States. Omnibus Budget Reconciliation Act of 1987. 2. Homes for the Aged—United States. 3. Geriatric Psychiatry—United States. 4. Health Policy—United States. 5. Mental Health Services—United States. 6. Nursing Homes—United States. WT 27.1 B619p 2000]
    RC451.4.N87 B57 2000
    618.97'689—dc21

                                            00-058137

ISBN : 978-0-7890-1219-7 (pbk)

CONTENTS

ABOUT THE AUTHOR

D. Peter Birkett, MD, is Director of Fellowship Training in geriatric psychiatry in the Columbia University/New York State program. His training was in the fields of geriatrics, internal medicine, neuropathology, and psychiatry. One of the first physicians to specialize in geriatric psychiatry, he served for 20 years as the medical director of a nursing home.

Dr. Birkett has published numerous research papers in the field of geriatric psychiatry. His most recent book was *The Psychiatry of Stroke*. He is a Fellow of the Royal College of Physicians of Canada, a Fellow of the Royal College of Psychiatrists of the United Kingdom, and a Member of the Royal College of Physicians of Edinburgh.

Introduction

Why are people put in nursing homes? Is the increase of nursing homes a bad thing? Can it go on? Who should care for the demented? How should long-term care be paid for? Many are puzzled by these questions.

State mental hospital populations have decreased; jail populations have increased; the numbers of homeless are rising; new kinds of residential institutions have developed; America is aging. These interrelated issues cannot be separated from psychiatry, although they may belong to policy and politics rather than clinical psychiatry.

This book, therefore, has a double target. It is particularly aimed at the practical needs of psychiatrists who work in nursing homes but raises questions that go beyond immediate practical issues. It is a broad survey of the new asylums, as well as a clinical handbook, and is meant for all who work with the elderly and chronically ill. A precise aim at a narrowly targeted audience would do an injustice to the subject. Nursing home patients have multiple problems, and those dealing with them come from many different backgrounds.

One result of casting a wide net for readers is that I have included material of a basic nature, meant to be useful for those who are venturing outside their own fields. This material includes simplified and dogmatic explanations of psychiatric issues. I hope those who are irritated by this will bear with me in the belief that the sin of too great a simplification is less than that of too great an obscurity.

I have also tried to tread the narrow line between the unreadable annotated bibliography and the unsupported expression of personal opinion. The factual information is, as far as possible, evidence-based, but in many areas objective quantified facts are lacking so that personal experience must be drawn upon. The experience is that of many years as medical director of a proprietary nursing home in the United States as well as purely psychiatric practice and work in other countries.

Case histories have been chosen to represent what is typical, rather than what is classical. Where these take the form of reports on my own cases, enough is altered to protect identities, but not enough to pretend that I solved every problem presented to me. It is more instructive to leave such loose ends untidily untied than tidily tied.

Updating the original edition has been more radical than I thought it would be. More changes have occurred than merely the advent of new psychotropic medications. Geriatric psychiatry has matured as a specialty; awareness of dementia as a psychiatric illness has increased; the tide of AIDS has crested in the United States and begun to turn; new legislation has been enacted; assisted living and HMOs have been introduced.

In the earliest part of the book, I shall play the Ghost of Christmas Past and survey the development of nursing homes and the events leading to enactment of the Omnibus Reconciliation Act of 1987 (OBRA). Then I will explain legal and administrative aspects, money matters, and how to deal with the red tape and form filling that so often threaten to strangle our efforts to help nursing home patients.

The next few chapters are broadly concerned with the people of the nursing home: the patients, the staff, and the families. These are considered in ways derived from sociology and anthropology.

Then comes consideration of the kinds of behavioral problems that are especially common in nursing home patients. These problems are categorized according to symptoms rather than diseases. This is not meant to question the validity of DSM and ICD diagnoses but to improve the practical usefulness of the advice given. The emphasis on nonmedication approaches is justified by the abundance of drug information now available from so many other sources.

Later sections are concerned with the medical/psychiatric interface so characteristic of the nursing home. Finally, I allow myself a wider perspective, and foretell the Christmases yet to come.

I shall use "he" when discussing conditions such as alcoholism and violence that are more common in males, and assume that the typical elderly nursing home patient is female.

PART I:
THE PLACES

Chapter 1

The History of Nursing Homes

Nursing homes in one guise or another had been around for many years before the 1960s.

Poorhouses, county homes, almshouses, and so forth have always existed in America. There were small homes for the aged financed by the residents' Social Security payments. There were privately run nursing homes that took those who could pay for as long as they could pay. The state hospitals contained large numbers of the elderly, and in many states these institutions were willing to accept all comers, including victims of purely physical chronic illness.

In one state hospital in Connecticut where I worked, several of the wards contained long rows of closely spaced beds. The occupants of these suffered from disabling physical illnesses. The most unfortunate, perhaps, were those who were of perfectly sound mind apart from the distress caused by their circumstances. They were put there to stay until they died.

The advent of large numbers of efficient, privately run, Medicaid-funded nursing homes saved thousands from such situations in the government-run hospitals. The 1950 amendments to the 1935 Social Security Act provided an increased level of funding for Old Age Assistance. These amendments included federal matching funds for medical services in nursing homes, although they excluded such matching funds to state and county mental hospitals (Kidder, 1999). The modern American nursing home resulted from the Medicaid and Medicare programs established in 1965. The standards for the homes were largely set by Medicare, although it was Medicaid that became largely responsible for their funding and rapid expansion in the 1970s. In 1970, 10 percent of the population was over sixty-five years old, and of these, 7 percent lived in such institutions as nursing homes, mental hospitals, and homes for the aged (Stotsky, 1972). By

1997, 1.6 million people lived in the nation's 17,168 nursing homes (Smith, 1998).

Medicaid was not intended to relieve states of the burden of caring for their mentally ill in the state hospitals. The law (Medicaid Transmittal, 1977) said that if over half the patients in a home were mentally ill then it should be designated as an Institution for Mental Disease (IMD). Guidelines were drawn up for the IMDs. Along with these guidelines went the stipulation that IMDs could not be supported by Medicaid. Naturally, no IMDs were set up (except for some in California).

The Community Mental Health Act of 1963 gave money to the states for psychiatry, but only for patients who were not in state hospitals. The states were supposed to go on paying for the state hospital patients out of state money. (There is some Medicaid and Medicare coverage in a state psychiatric hospital, but this is very limited and restricted.)

OMNIBUS RECONCILIATION ACT OF 1987

Hard-pressed though the state treasurers were, the feds remained suspicious that states were using some of this nursing home money to subsidize their state mental health systems. Evidence accumulated that, in spite of where federal law said the mentally ill belonged, they were put into nursing homes so that the money for their care would come from Medicaid, not out of the state mental health funds. This was one of the considerations that led to the new provisions of OBRA, the Omnibus Reconciliation Act of 1987. (OBRA Acts are passed frequently, but anyone who refers to "OBRA" in talking about nursing homes means the act of 1987.)

These new provisions made a further effort to keep the mentally ill out of the nursing homes. Compliance with OBRA occupied the attention of those concerned with nursing home care for several years thereafter. Nursing homes were not prohibited from taking psychiatric patients. It was merely mandated that the patient was to get active treatment (the term "active treatment" for mental illness was later replaced by "specialized services") and that treatment was not covered by Medicaid. Thus, it was up to the nursing homes to ensure that they did not get stuck with psychiatric patients.

The Final Rule issued by the Health Care Financing Administration (HCFA) in September 1991, made a distinction between "rehabilitative services" for mental illness (which the nursing home is supposed to be able to provide) and "specialized services" (which are "outside the scope of nursing facility mental health services.") An example of the former would be treatment for mild depression. Making fine Talmudic distinctions of this kind can be of practical importance in the nursing home business because of the need to comply with such government regulations. The 1991 Final Rule said, "We believe that specialized services can only be ordinarily delivered in the NF setting with difficulty because the overall level of services in NFs is not as intense as needed to address these needs." The Rule went on to say that a state's Preadmission Screening and Annual Resident Review (PASARR) program (see Chapter 2) could determine that an individual with mental illness or mental retardation "may enter or continue to reside in the NF, even though he or she needs specialized services" but warned that "if the individual does so, then the State must provide or arrange for the provision of additional services to raise the level of intensity of services to the level needed by the resident" (Comment on §483.45(a)).

OBRA Exemptions

Several exemptions provided loopholes for admission of the mentally ill. For example, presence of a medical illness may get a mentally ill patient into a nursing home. This "medical override" can come into effect if the patient is terminally ill or comatose, is convalescing from a recoverable condition following hospitalization, or has severe lung or heart disease, or certain progressive neurological diseases. Another exemption is for dementia due to Alzheimer's disease and related conditions, but if the diagnosis of dementia is made, it has to be substantiated by investigations and consultations.

It is difficult to diagnose dementia in the mentally retarded. For this reason Alzheimer's disease is not given any specific mention in the sections on mental retardation (*Federal Register,* 1989). The prohibition against admission to a nursing home presumably applies to the mentally retarded even if "dementia" is also diagnosed. However, the "ICF-MR" category (see Chapter 11) has been retained so that

Medicaid can fund care for the mentally retarded in certain institutions.

OBRA and Psychotropic Medication

OBRA took a definite stand against antipsychotic drugs and recommended that they should be used only to treat a specific condition. It recommended attempts to reduce their use, such as trials of dose reduction and of stopping the drugs (drug holidays) and substitution of behavioral programming.

The federal law apparently stigmatized the use of psychotropic drugs as "chemical restraint," which aroused the indignation of ardent psychopharmacologists. The exact wording as published in the *Federal Register,* Vol 54, February 2, 1989, was:

> § 483.13 Level A requirement: Resident behavior and facility practices.
> (a) Level B requirement: Restraints. The resident has the right to be free from any physical restraint imposed or psychoactive drug administered for purposes of discipline or convenience, and not required to treat the resident's medical symptoms.

Some further federal regulations are as follows:

> Code of Federal Regulations; 483.25(1)
> (2) Antipsychotic drugs. Based on a comprehensive assessment of a resident, the facility must ensure that:
> (i) Residents who have not used anti-psychotic drugs are not given these drugs unless antipsychotic drug therapy is necessary to treat a specific condition as diagnosed and documented in the clinical record and
> (ii) Residents who use antipsychotic drugs receive gradual dose reductions, and behavioral interventions, unless clinically contraindicated, in an effort to discontinue these drugs.

This wording did allow for a nonpsychiatric physician or other practitioner to do the documentation, but in practice, for better or for worse, most nursing homes find it easiest to get a psychiatrist to meet the requirements.

Section 1819 and 1919(c)(1)(D) of OBRA 1987 says that "psychopharmacologic drugs" can be prescribed "only if, at least annually, an independent external consultant reviews the appropriateness of the drug plan of each resident receiving such drugs." The qualifications of this external consultant have not been defined (Kidder, 1999). The problems arising from these drug use regulations are further discussed in Chapter 10.

Did OBRA Improve Things?

The start-up date for the OBRA requirements was October 1, 1990, but it took a long time for anything to happen. The implementation rules and "interpretive guidelines" are the work of the Health Care Financing Administration (HCFA) in the Department of Health and Human Services, which performs for mystic writings of Congress the functions of Daniel before Nebuchadnezzar. Some of these rules and guidelines continue to be changed.

In the next two chapters, we shall examine some of the mountains of paperwork the regulations produced and the evidence that they failed to reduce the number of mentally ill in the nursing homes.

Chapter 2

Paper, Paper, Paper

A set of nursing home records may be several inches thick, and the staff will complain that most of their time is spent on paperwork. To what extent is psychiatry responsible for this, and what can psychiatry do about it?

Some of the work is psychiatric. Nursing home charts are required by law to have a comprehensive assessment of the patient's psychosocial needs on the chart. This is usually done by the social worker (see Chapter 8), although that is not mandatory. It is supposed to document such things as outside contacts, frequency of visitors, use of free time, preinstitutional hobbies and interests, participation in activities, communication, orientation, and behavior. This is often the most useful document in the chart for telling what is really going on with the patient, and why he or she is in a nursing home. It is more extensive and more legible than the doctor's history and physical examination (which, to be fair to my colleagues, has to be on the chart within two days of admission, whereas the social worker has two weeks from the admission date).

CARE PLANS

A comprehensive care plan, mandated by OBRA and already in place as a requirement in many states, is supposed to be developed after the comprehensive assessment and updated at intervals. It must be prepared by an interdisciplinary team that includes the attending physician, a registered nurse, and other staff, plus, if possible, the patient or the patient's representative.

Sometimes a multidisciplinary care plan is produced without a genuine meeting ever taking place. The plan contains formulaic phrases, and is passed around for different professionals to sign, none of whom had any real input. It is then kept for a required period of time and discarded without having served a useful purpose.

A multidisciplinary care plan (MCP) can be useful and can actually save time if correctly carried out. Circumventing it can increase work. Once the plan is agreed to at the meeting, it can be referenced to avoid prolonged misunderstandings and arguments at the nursing station or over the telephone. Formulating care plans requires mastery of a certain jargon that may be unfamiliar to the medically trained. Traditional medical care planning consisted of the patient's complaints or symptoms, followed by a diagnosis and then by treatment, hopefully based on the diagnosis. Currently, fashionable care planning consists of problems, goals, and interventions. It always sounds good to interpolate the magic phrases "evidenced by" and "related to," and to use MCP terminology. The "problem" can be stated in various ways. It can be a disability such as inability to walk, or a symptom such as pain, or a medical diagnosis such as "hip fracture."

Nursing staff often have trouble complying with documentation of behavioral interventions for problem behaviors (Llorente et al., 1998):

> An eighteen-year-old mentally retarded diplegic cerebral palsy victim with no understandable speech was showing signs of agitation and distress. At a care plan meeting staff members said, "We try to show him we love him. Some of us come in to see him on our time off. We bring him toys and pictures to look at. We hug him and talk to him." However, they said they could not document a care plan because, "There's nothing we can do for him."

ACRONYMS

RUG, RAP, MDS, and RAI stand for Resource Utilization Group, Resident Assessment Protocol, Minimum Data Set, and Resident Assessment Instrument. MDS and RAP are long and involved questionnaires about the patient.

The MDS "triggers" the RAP. MDS and RAP (plus some others) taken together comprise the RAI. (Outcome Assessment Information

Set [OASIS] is the home care equivalent of the RAI.) Digits and signs may be added to these after the manner of software manufacturers, as new and improved versions are introduced, so that RAI has become RAI2. PASARR (Preadmission Screening and Annual Resident Review) is done on every potential resident whose MDS shows evidence of mental illness other than dementia. If such evidence is confirmed the review is to be repeated annually.

Resource Utilization Group (RUG)

The RAI determines the RUG classification, which decides if the nursing home can get paid for the patient. The RUG classification system is of the "sicker the better" type. Mental status enters very little into the equation (Beckwith, 1998).

Minimum Data Set (MDS)

It used to be possible for a patient to be in a nursing home with a diagnosis listed as congestive heart failure when the real problems were incontinence and inability to walk. The record stated that the patient had "CHF due to ASHD (congestive heart failure due to arteriosclerotic heart disease)" and that the treatment was cardiac medication.

This still occurs to a large extent, reflecting the concept of the nursing home as a kind, albeit an inferior kind, of general hospital. The new Minimum Data Set was intended to give a more rational and comprehensive picture of the patient.

The MDS is in many ways a superb instrument. It was devised by the prestigious Institute of Medicine (a quasigovernmental organization appointed by the National Academy of Science to which the federal government gives money to conduct inquiries and issue reports). It possesses excellent psychometric properties of reliability and validity (Lawton et al., 1998; Casten et al., 1998) and is even used outside the United States (Finne-Soveri and Tilvis, 1998).

It is a monument of intellectual achievement but resembles other monuments erected by governments, such as the pyramids, in taking up a lot of the taxpayers' time and money. The 284 beautifully crafted items are to be completed by the nurse in charge of each unit (within fourteen days of admission and then once a year). The nurse must call upon the aides, social workers, doctors, and activities staff to get the information needed to complete the form. Some nurses believe their time could be better spent.

The patient has ample leisure but does not get asked to help complete the MDS. The MDS assumes, as Kane (1998) points out, that the patients are incapable of giving direct input into a document supposedly designed to find out if they are getting good care. Other criticisms have been made, and some commentators have found that the form is time-consuming and contains many antiquated ideas.

Resident Assessment Protocol (RAP)

The MDS involves answering many questions about every aspect of the patient. If an answer indicates a problem area, then a more detailed set of questions about that area is indicated. This more detailed and focused inquiry is a RAP. For example, one of the questions is about weight gain or loss. "Has the patient gained or lost 5 percent in weight in the last thirty days?" If the answer is yes, then this triggers a RAP, which involves a more detailed assessment of the patient's nutritional status and formulation of a plan to do something about it. Here again, the patients have little input about what they think is wrong. For example, as Engle (1998) points out, there are no RAP triggers for pain or dyspnea.

Preadmission Screening and Annual Resident Review (PASARR)

Preadmission Screening and Annual Resident Review (PASARR) is the form that is supposed to determine whether someone is sane enough to be in a nursing home. It was devised with the aim of not admitting the mentally ill (Borson et al., 1997) as part of the OBRA '87 legislation. States were allowed to devise their own versions of PASARR. The law (as formulated by HCFA a "Final Rule" of September 1991) stated that if a state PASARR allowed admission to a nursing home of a patient who needs psychiatric "specialized services," then the state is obliged to provide them.

Much paperwork in nursing homes has resulted from a tendency to fight paper with paper. Examination of a six-inch thick chart will often reveal that many of the forms and duplications are generated within the nursing home itself, often resulting from a misunderstanding of regulatory requirements. Fear of "the State" and "the inspectors" can generate superstitions about what they need. For example, if a state agency specifies that a patient's chart must contain a "mental status and psychosocial summary," then some institutions will insist that a separate piece of paper must be included labeled "mental status and psychosocial summary." Often a fresh form will be created for this purpose, and staff will be told that the state requires this form. Psychiatric nurses are sometimes employed to fill out such papers but then find they have little further input into the patient care. Once a new form or set of paperwork has been created, it becomes very difficult to get rid of it. One reason for this is that any change creates extra work. The unfamiliar occupies more time even if it is shorter.

Chapter 3

The New Asylums?

The number of beds in public mental hospitals decreased from 560,000 in 1955 to 80,000 in 1995. As the population of state mental hospitals in the United States has decreased, the population of nursing homes has increased. The symmetry of this statistic suggests that the so-called deinstitutionalization of the mentally disordered is really a reinstitutionalization, with the population being incarcerated in nursing homes instead of mental hospitals. Some authorities regarded it as self-evident that the state hospital population has shifted to the nursing homes. To quote an editorial by Dr. John Talbott in *Hospital and Community Psychiatry* (1988, p. 115): "Over the past thirty-three years, state hospitals have shrunk to a third of their former size, and the number of nursing homes has more than trebled. Coincidence? Hardly."

THE HOMELESS AND THE JAILED

Other candidates vie for the title of the new asylums. For example, the population of U.S. jails totaled 200,000 in 1972, but increased to 2,000,000 in 1996 (Bureau of Justice Statistics Jail Statistics <www.ojp.usdoj.gov/bjs/jails>). The number of the homeless has also increased, although to what extent this population varies depends on who is doing the counting. Also, as we shall see, many kinds of transitional residences accommodate the mentally ill.

DEINSTITUTIONALIZATION
AND TRANSINSTITUTIONALIZATION

Opinions differ as to whether new medications or new theories led to the decline of the state hospitals. Whether by coincidence or design, the process of transfer to the nursing homes started soon after

17

the Community Mental Health Center Act of 1963. This provided the states with funding for programs that were supposed to help the severely ill who had been in the state hospitals. Federally funded community mental health centers were set up and the states tried to stop admitting anyone to their state-funded hospitals. The states took the money and ran, setting up big, beautiful community mental health centers, which employed many people. They also tried to stop admissions to their state hospitals, but this was through a process of barring the doors rather than curing the patients before they were sick enough to need admission.

All this was happening at a time when the effectiveness of medications in helping the mentally ill was beginning to dawn on the public. Fluctuating political fashions were also at work. In Italy, for example, Law 180 was passed in 1978, largely at the instigation of Franco Basaglia, a Marxist follower of Ronald Laing and Thomas Szasz, and Italian mental hospitals and inpatient psychiatric facilities were abruptly closed by government decree.

The Initial Surge of Transfers

At first the idea of shifting patients from mental hospitals to nursing homes was regarded with equanimity (at least by those in medical authority). There was no doubt that it was happening and little question about whether it should be happening.

Redlich and Kellert (1978) revisited data from the classical 1958 study of Hollingshead and Redlich. They stated unequivocally that the fall in state hospital populations was due to discharge of patients to nursing homes. The primary reason for this shift was to transfer the financial burden from the state-financed mental hospitals to federal funding. "The nursing home appeared to have significantly reduced a major cost burden on the mental health system (at least 50 percent of the cost of custodial care)"(p. 24). They found that "in 1950 chronic patients filled the back wards of the state hospital, but by 1975 most of them had been discharged to nursing homes" and "in 1975 approximately half of the aged chronically ill patients discharged from the state hospital were referred to nursing homes" (Redlich and Kellert, 1978, p. 24). Between 1950 and 1970 the mean age for inpatients in the state facilities was over fifty, and by 1975 it was approximately forty. They stated that the proportion of patients with "senile/organic" disorders in the state hospitals decreased from 18 percent in 1950 to 1 percent in 1975.

This study was limited to an area around New Haven, Connecticut, which may have been atypical of the United States as a whole. However, the depth and thoroughness of the study is unrivaled in terms of comparing the situation in 1950 with that in 1975. It must be remembered that up until the 1960s, many state hospitals literally functioned as asylums and admitted the chronically ill, even without any diagnosed mental illness.

The Backlash

Further changes occurred in the late 1970s and the 1980s. Many nursing homes stopped admitting patients from state hospitals because the state hospitals refused to take the patients back when they became acutely psychotic. The policy (if there was such a policy) of putting the mentally ill in nursing homes began to be questioned.

Schmidt and colleagues (1977) were among the first to be alarmed by the supposed shift of the mentally ill to the nursing homes. The title of their paper was "The Mentally Ill in Nursing Homes: New Back Wards in the Community," which suggests their theme. They used Medicaid data from Utah nursing homes and found that a third of the residents had a psychiatric diagnosis and that more than half of these were psychotic. The psychotic residents actually received fewer psychoactive drugs than did the nonpsychotic residents.

Surveys

Several studies were subsequently conducted to determine whether the mentally ill had in fact been shifted to the nursing homes. The studies were done by examining the incidence of mental disorder in these institutions.

Teeter, Garetz, and Miller (1976) studied a random sample of the population of two proprietary nursing homes in the Midwest. Patients and staff were interviewed by a social worker, using a rating scale for cognitive function in addition to diagnostic interviews. Charts were reviewed by a psychiatrist. Eighty-five percent had major psychiatric disorders, of whom less than a third had recorded psychiatric diagnoses.

Rovner and colleagues (1986) studied in detail fifty residents chosen at random from the population of one proprietary nursing home in Baltimore. Residents were mainly widowed, female, and white, with a mean age of eighty-three. Almost all had a major psychiatric diagnosis, most often dementia. Most had delusions or hallucinations. They concluded that the nursing home was "in reality a long-term psychiatric facility without its having the usual trained personnel and treatment approaches found in psychiatric hospitals."

Estimates of the number of mentally ill in nursing homes continued to vary considerably, from as low as 30 percent (if this is low) to as high as 85 percent (Beardsley et al., 1989). More cases were found by researchers who used psychometric scales and conducted direct patient interviews in their surveys. Linn and colleagues (1985) found that, even allowing for varying ascertainment methods, there was a true increase. The findings of Rovner et al. (1986) in Maryland were replicated by Tariot et al. (1993) in New York.

Schizophrenia in the Nursing Home

Such studies certainly showed a high incidence of mental disorder in the nursing homes. However, the kinds of mental disorder that filled the nursing homes were different from those of the mental hospitals. The nursing home patients were largely demented or depressed, whereas the mental hospital patients were schizophrenic.

Could some of the allegedly demented nursing home residents be former schizophrenics? Certainly a large group of nursing home patients are labeled as demented and simply do not communicate enough for any diagnosis to be established. Some surveys may include these as demented and missing ex-schizophrenics. Inability to communicate leads to prolonged institutionalization of schizophrenic patients. The articulate and paranoid talk their way out of institutions, no matter how dangerous; the incoherent and hebephrenic stay in, no matter how harmless.

This is challenged by our knowledge of the natural history of aging schizophrenics. They have no particular tendency to develop into noncommunicators who could be labeled as demented. Another fact about the natural history of schizophrenia is that it leads to early death. Its victims, especially males, do not live long enough to enter nursing homes in old age.

Surveys of the present populations of state hospitals do not suggest that they got rid of their elderly or physically frail. Their present inpatient population is largely composed of the very old. It looks more as if they reduced their censuses (and the burden on state budgets) by discharging or turning away young and physically fit psychotics, who then ended up in the streets, the jails, or in the board and care homes.

The elderly remaining in the state hospitals have mostly been admitted at young ages with a diagnosis of paranoid schizophrenia. Those who enter the state hospitals in old age with a paranoid diagnosis often respond to treatment and are discharged (Goodman and Siegel, 1986)

In solving the mystery by investigating the history of present nursing home populations, we encounter the same difficulty faced by the framers of OBRA: deciding who is a former mental hospital patient. How far back do we go, and how deep do we dig? Do we count those who were in psychiatric units in general hospitals, or those who were in county hospitals, or those who had a brief psychotic episode many years previously? Previous histories of mental hospitalization are often deliberately or accidentally concealed on admission to a nursing home. Over the years I have often encountered old friends in the nursing homes whom I remembered from my days in the local state hospital. Their written records contained no trace of their psychiatric history.

Probably, taking various surveys together, about 10 percent of nursing home patients suffer from schizophrenia (Citrome, 1998) and about 200,000 patients with chronic schizophrenia have been transferred from American mental hospitals to nursing homes (Harvey et al., 1998). (These figures do not include the board and care homes, which contain large numbers of the younger mentally ill.) Most sources of error in counting are likely to produce underestimation rather than overestimation. Schizophrenia in poorly communicating patients is likely to be mistaken for dementia. The requirements for admission to nursing homes are such that those filling out the application forms are induced to conceal histories of psychosis. Doctors and discharge planners who want to get patients into nursing homes and then are confronted with a form that says the patient will not be admitted with a primary diagnosis of psychosis other than dementia are liable to make the diagnostic discovery that their patient does not have a primary diagnosis of psychosis other than dementia. (The issue of schizophrenia in the nursing home is further discussed in Chapter 12.)

Were They Better Off in the Nursing Homes?

A different approach was to suggest that, even if the mentally ill had been put into nursing homes, they might be just as well off there as in the state mental hospitals. This certainly seemed to be true for some of the physically ill. Indeed, the American Psychiatric Association (1998) conjured up a vision of psychotic patients clamoring for their right to be put in nursing homes and being foiled by legislation that stigmatized them as risky.

Shadish and Bootzin (1981) said that the mentally ill had indeed been displaced into the nursing homes, but suggested that this might be beneficial because they needed asylum anyway. The government should admit its mistake in attempting deinstitutionalization, and should make the best of a bad job by providing psychiatric services to those in the nursing homes. Loebel and Rabitt (1988, pp. 997-998) claimed that "with relatively brief and inexpensive interventions, psychosocial components can be added . . . polypharmacy avoided, depression and confusion treated, and autonomy enhanced" in the nursing home.

Carling (1981), a former federal policymaking official, took issue with Shadish and Bootzin, and said that the government should do no such thing, and that the mentally ill should be kept out of nursing homes.

Such disputes led to attempts to determine how badly off the mentally ill were in nursing homes. The most influential of these was the Veterans Administration Cooperative Study (Linn et al., 1985). The results can be viewed in several ways. Essentially the study took two matched groups of patients in VA hospitals and discharged some of them to nursing homes and sent some of them into other psychiatric hospital units. The group placed in nursing homes did worse in every measurable way. This applied even to those without functional psychosis. Demented patients did better in psychiatric hospital settings than in nursing homes. Schizophrenic patients placed in nursing homes tended to become dependent and indistinguishable, functionally, from the demented. They apparently became conditioned to having things done for them and stopped doing things for themselves.

However, the cost of caring for each patient for a year in a psychiatric hospital at that time was $31,000, and the cost in the nursing homes was $20,000. It could be argued that for an extra $11,000 the nursing homes could have provided comparable care.

Loopholes

OBRA '87 was enacted in the face of evidence that nursing homes were really miniature mental hospitals. The bill was supported by patient advocacy groups such as the National Mental Health Association. The law was framed to suggest that the intention was to improve treatment of the mentally ill, by specifying that they could be admitted only to an institution that provided active care.

Most interpreted this to mean that the mentally ill could not be admitted to nursing homes. The law seemed to imply, however, that the demented could be admitted to nursing homes, and also that the mentally ill could be admitted if mental illness was not their primary diagnosis. This dementia exemption and the medical override became a wide-open door.

To a large extent, the states are circumventing the requirements about keeping the mentally ill out of nursing homes. In some cases this is done openly, by state requirements that are in contravention of OBRA, or in some cases by interpretations that bend the rules. Nondemented mentally ill patients who might actually be better off in lesser care facilities continue to be misplaced into nursing homes (Snowden, Piacitelli and Koepsell, 1998). The nursing homes continue to contain the grossly psychotic and the states show little inclination to provide services for them.

Chapter 4

What Is a Nursing Home?

Not all the institutions in which the sick are housed are hospitals or nursing homes. It is important for all health practitioners to be aware of the status of institutions in which their patients live. I have known a hospital patient to be discharged to a boarding house after surgery with instructions given to the staff to keep the patient in bed, change dressings, and observe for complications. The hospital staff were under the impression that he was being transferred to a "nursing home."

A knowledge of the other types of residential facilities is useful to those who provide psychosocial services of any kind within the nursing homes. It is especially essential for those who are involved in the placement of patients. Deciding where a sick person belongs within the spectrum of care is becoming an increasingly professional activity.

SKILLED NURSING FACILITIES
AND INTERMEDIATE CARE FACILITIES

The term "nursing home" seldom appears in federal legislation. The Medicare Act contains a definition of a "skilled nursing facility" and the Medicaid Act contains a somewhat broader definition of a "nursing facility" (Braun, 1998). Nursing facilities all provide care by registered nurses. They maintain records and have an attending physician designated for each patient in the same way a regular hospital does. A nursing home has to provide round-the-clock nursing. There must be at least a licensed practical nurse (LPN) available twenty-four hours a day, every day, and a registered nurse for eight hours a day, seven days a week.

A Skilled Nursing Facility (SNF) is a nursing facility that can, in certain circumstances and for a limited time, be reimbursed by Medicare, not Medicaid, and can provide a level of care almost equivalent to that of a hospital. Most nursing facilities qualify as being SNFs. Earlier legislation (the "Miller Amendments" promulgated as federal standards in 1971) provided for another level of care called an Intermediate Care Facility (ICF). Both are commonly called nursing homes. The ICF was intended to provide a rather less intense level of care, although still with RN or LPN availability twenty-four hours a day. In some jurisdictions the ICFs were called Health Related Facilities (HRFs). The ICF then virtually disappeared, with one exception, which concerns the mentally retarded (see Chapter 11).

BOARD AND CARE FACILITIES

Theoretically at least, OBRA '87 meant that many patients with mental illness formerly placed in nursing homes would no longer be eligible for such placement. The nursing homes themselves would have been faced with the necessity of, to put it bluntly, getting rid of them, or providing them with active psychiatric treatment which would not be reimbursed by Medicaid. This may have been a stimulus to the increase of unregulated lesser care facilities, although many other factors were at work, ranging from the use of new medications to changes in America's vacation habits.

The lesser care facilities are a heterogeneous set of living places, probably because there are no federal guidelines defining or limiting them. They are so heterogeneous that it is difficult to obtain accurate statistics about them, but they are probably the primary place in which the former state mental hospital patients are found. Essentially, they differ from the nursing homes in not being reimbursed by Medicaid, and not having any nursing staff. Matters of nomenclature have not been made any easier by changes over the course of time and variations between states.

These homes vary from having several hundred residents to one or two, and this makes any generalization about them difficult, because the lower end includes completely informal arrangements where someone looks after one or two disabled or elderly people and is paid "off the books." They usually provide some supervision of medication and most of them do not insist that residents are able to walk (Hames et al., 1995; Stoecklin et al., 1998).

Some of the names given to such homes are: residential care facilities, board and care, community care homes, personal care homes, domiciliary care homes, supervisory care homes, sheltered care facilities, adult foster care, family homes, group homes, transitional living facilities, halfway houses, homes for the aged, continuing care facilities, and adult homes. Assisted (or assistive) living is a separate category in some states. Even within a state the facilities may be referred to by one name in official regulations and have another colloquial name. The amount of licensing and regulation may vary considerably, and the same name may have various meanings in different states (Benjamin and Newcomer, 1986). In 1993, the United States had about 34,000 licensed board and care facilities with 613,000 beds, as well as many unlicensed facilities. Most of the residents were elderly—about 80 percent over age sixty-five—and a third of them were on psychotropic drugs. Eight percent had been previously psychiatrically hospitalized (Spore at al., 1995).

A New York group home is a regular house in a residential area, purchased by the state at market prices, and staffed around the clock by state employees, or by employees of an agency under contract to the state. Most of these house the young mentally retarded.

Adult foster care and family homes are often informal arrangements for the aged or mentally ill to live with an unrelated family. In some states these are supervised and subsidized.

SROs (single room occupancy hotels) are what their name suggests: very cheap hotels. The occupants are responsible for paying their own rent to the landlord, and are not under any kind of supervision. In many cases, a social service department, faced with a homeless family and no place to put them, pays the regular rent on a hotel or motel room for them. Hotels that can find no way to keep such clients out (and there is no legal way) find themselves rapidly on the skids and become known as "welfare hotels." In these "welfare hotels" the rent is paid by the social service department (welfare) directly to the landlord.

The Adult Care Homes of New York State (see Assisted Living, p. 31) may contain several hundred residents. Many of these started off as hotels to which middle-class people might go on vacation. As the suburbs surrounded them, and their former clientele went to Aspen or Cape Cod for vacations, they became what are commonly thought of as "old people's homes" or "rest homes." They took in, as permanent residents, nice old people who paid their own way. As the supply of these nice old people began to dwindle, and as the nice old people became less nice because they were demented or ill, the state hospitals began discharging their clients to these places. In many cases, psychotic patients neglected themselves or behaved in ways that alarmed the public, and regulations were made tighter and tighter, including a modicum of psychiatric training for the adminis-trators.

"Rest homes" in Massachusetts provide at least four hours of con-sultation by a licensed nurse per forty-bed unit per month, and physi-cal examinations are required on admission, then once every six months (Avorn et al., 1989; Bowland, 1989).

All of these institutions are distinguished from nursing homes by the method of payment. They are not paid for by Medicaid. Unless a private arrangement is made, the board and care home (adult home, rest home, or sheltered care facility) is usually paid for by the resi-dent's Social Security checks, Supplementary Security Income (SSI) checks, or welfare checks. (SSI is a kind of federal welfare paid to those disabled who never made Social Security payments and to those on Social Security whose income is not enough to meet their needs.) This is often barely enough to cover the rental of accommodations in areas of expensive real estate. Indeed, the price of real estate is driv-ing the board and care home operators out of business in the metro-politan areas. Providing food and room maintenance on top of this rental factor can become difficult, and providing further services im-possible. Thus, these patients are often unsatisfactorily lodged and the tendency is to look for someone to blame. Mental health profession-als who are unfamiliar with these homes tend to expect too much of them.

Probably over a million residents live in such homes, but the number is hard to determine because of differences in definition (Benjamin and Newcomer, 1986). The rather limited data on psychiatric drug use and other issues in these homes has been reviewed by Avorn et al. (1989) and indicates that about a third of the residents may be former state hospital patients, and over half of them are on psychotropic drugs.

Many of the former state hospital patients present formidable man-agement difficulties. In some cases the transition is smooth. For ex-ample, the patient may be a chronic schizophrenic without drug or alcohol problems or physical illness, who takes medication and attends a day program organized by a community mental health center, with the community mental health center also providing emergency psychiatric services. This smooth transition is by no means the rule, however.

The younger patients often smoke marijuana, drink alcohol, and take various other drugs. Not only do these have some adverse direct effect on their brain, but also they use up the money provided for their support, thus neglecting their clothing and grooming.

Cigarettes are perhaps an even bigger problem than drugs and alcohol. The schizophrenics seem to be the last holdouts in the decline of cigarette smokers in America and Britain (Kelly and McCreadie, 1999). Many of them spend much time in the acute care general hospital being treated for respiratory ailments, peptic ulcers, and other tobacco-related illnesses. They have a high mortality rate.

The admixture of nonpsychiatric medical illnesses progresses among the older residents. These older residents include some of the traditional types of residents of old people's homes, but now also include the elderly psychotic. These individuals may often have serious medical illnesses that they neglect, yet they seek medical attention for very minor conditions. A patient with a large lump in her breast, for example, may persistently demand cough medicine.

It is usually hard to arrange for a direct transfer from a board and care home to a nursing home. The nursing homes run with 100 percent capacity, and candidates for admission, therefore, must be put on a waiting list. The typically approved mechanism is for a form to be completed by a health care professional who scores the level of care needed (see Chapter 2). The home must find such professionals and figure out when they can come, and how they are to be paid. If the "score" allows nursing home placement, the adult home is now automatically in violation of the state code and must document efforts to place the patient, using its own limited clerical resources. The most common solution to this doctor's dilemma is to place the patient in an acute care general hospital. Such hospitalization is often the only way to get the patient to a higher level of care. Having the waiting client unsuitably placed in a hospital, while awaiting a nursing home bed, is an annoyance. However, it is not as bad as having the client in a board and care home. The hospital that wants to discharge a patient can use the help of battalions of skilled discharge planners, whereas the board and care homes are poorly staffed, even for the function of removing residents when they want to.

Although it is easy to list the negatives of these places, professionals should avoid an antagonistic attitude toward them. On the whole, those who staff them do a remarkably good job for the money they receive. Good communication is the key to dealing with them, whatever the defects of the system. Everyone involved with community mental health should become familiar with the homes in their area, and get to know the staff and the patients.

SECTION 8 HOUSING

Senior Citizen Housing built under the 1974 Housing Act (often called Section 8 or Section 202 Housing) is housing built by a private builder (or charitable organization) with rents that are federally subsidized to the extent that they exceed 25 percent of the tenant's income. The legislation was meant to help those with limited funds but many of the residents come from affluent backgrounds. Quite often residents have moved out from run-down, inner-city areas to be closer to their families who have moved to the suburbs. Section 8 tenants must be either over sixty-five or disabled. A psychiatric disability could, in theory, qualify, but the hurdles to application are such that psychiatric patients rarely get these apartments. The most common types of mental illness found in these residents are late-life onset, occurring after the patients moved in, such as dementia and certain kinds of paranoia and depression.

HOME CARE AGENCIES

Home care agencies and visiting nurse associations were originally established to provide care in patients' homes employing nurses, home aides, and a variable assortment of health care providers. Home care was at one time thought to be a money saver but it is probably an expensive proposition when professionals are required to make house calls. Under certain circumstances Medicare and Medicaid will pay. Medicare can pay for services of a skilled nursing nature by a registered nurse on a time-limited basis. Medicaid is more flexible. A limitation on funding for home care for psychiatric illness required eligibility to be limited to the homebound. Many psychiatric patients do not meet this requirement.

Some home care agencies now provide services to patients in board and care residences. The funding agencies regard such patients as being in their own homes. When the board and care residence is large, the agency may maintain a presence in the building. The result is a hybrid level of care in which it is uncertain who is responsible for what.

ASSISTED LIVING

Assisted living is an up-market version of the board and care facility. In some ways it represents reemergence of the old "HRF" and "ICF" categories. Even for government officials and for experts on aging, deciding just what "assisted living" is can be confusing (Rimer, 1999). Four states, Alabama, Rhode Island, South Dakota, and Wyoming, use "assisted living" and "board and care" interchangeably. In other states, assisted living is designated in ways that allow the home to admit sicker patients and provide more health services. Thirty-five states currently provide Medicaid reimbursement or plan to do so. This Medicaid reimbursement can be made under a "1913c waiver" out of money that the state would otherwise spend on nursing home care. The average annual cost is $24,433 (*Provider,* 1998).

According to the American Association of Retired Persons (1999), "An assisted living facility is generally defined as a residential setting that provides or coordinates personal care services, 24-hour supervision, scheduled and unscheduled assistance, social activities, and some health related services." By this definition, several types of board and care residences, such as the New York adult homes, the Massachussetts level IV residential care facilities, the California residential care facilities, the Florida adult congregate living facilities, and the New Jersey type C and D boarding houses would qualify, but the same states also contain other residences designated as assisted living.

The average resident is eighty-three years old, female, ambulatory, and needs some help with activities of daily living. Twenty percent are incontinent to some degree. Almost half are demented, about 11 percent severely so (Vickery, 1998). Compared with other board and care home occupants, they are older and richer and less likely to suffer from schizophrenia or drug addiction or to have been in a state hospital.

It is possible that the recent increase in assisted living will reduce the numbers in the other board and care facilities, but statistics are difficult to obtain owing to the variable definitions. Probably about 600,000 individuals live in assisted care.

MIXED-LEVEL RETIREMENT COMMUNITIES

Sometimes board and care facilities exist on the same premises as nursing facilities. Such institutions were originally devised with the idea of providing a smooth pathway to the grave. Those who were admitted were to relinquish all their money and be cared for until they died. They signed agreements with a retirement community to provide lifetime care including nursing home care. They would usually give the institution several hundred thousand dollars and also pay from $500 to $2,000 a month (Pynoos, 1999). Such agreements have run into conflict with federal regulations governing who can be admitted to a nursing home, and special legislation has been enacted in some states. Standards for Continuing Care Retirement Communities (CCRCs) in New York were established by the Long-Term Care Integration and Finance Act of 1997. These provide independent living units, room and board, and limited health care benefits, including a minimum of sixty days of nursing facility care. The fate of those who become mentally ill, and who therefore do not qualify for nursing home admission under PASARR, is not yet clear.

Chapter 5

How the Homes Are Paid

Most (about 75 percent) nursing homes are privately owned, usually designated as "proprietary" or "for-profit," although they may be losing money. The rest are tax-exempt and may be run by government agencies or be "voluntary" and run by churches (5 percent) or other groups. Because they were designed to make money, the tendency has been to regard the "for-profits" as the bad guys, and they have been the subjects of exposure in the anti-nursing home diatribes. However, the tightness of government regulation and the way the money is distributed now evens out most differences.

Many nursing homes are owned by large chains whose managements are highly professional businesspeople. In some cases the actual ownership may be obscure. One person or group may own the business and rent the building. The owners of the building, in turn, may not own it outright but are paying off a mortgage. The mortgage holder may be a bank or another business group. (The business owners may also be paying off a note to a former owner of the business.) If the home is "voluntary," the ownership may be represented by a board of trustees.

The Veterans Administration has three separate nursing home programs. Nursing homes may be run directly by the VA, or the VA may fund placement in privately run nursing homes, or the VA may join with a state to fund nursing homes.

MEDICAID AND MEDICARE

Most nursing home stays are paid for by Medicaid, which is a mixture of state and federal funds. Medicare Part B pays for the doctors and for certain laboratory and other costs (see Balanced Budget Amendment, p. 36). Medicare Part B will pay for one doctor's visit per month, regardless of how the patient is doing. Further visits have to be "justified," and this justification is often a source of dispute and discontent. Nursing home patients must be seen by a doctor within thirty days of admission. After that, the visit frequency depends on state requirements and what Medicare will pay for.

Some of the money for nursing homes (about 10 percent) comes from Medicare Part A. Medicare Part A usually only pays for hospital care. Skilled nursing facility beds can, under certain narrowly defined circumstances, be reimbursed by Medicare rather than Medicaid. In effect, this (rather more generous) reimbursement is for patients just discharged from a hospital, although the requirements are complicated and have changed from time to time (Agronin, 1998). Patients discharged from a psychiatric hospital or general hospital psychiatric unit are excluded from this coverage.

THE "SPEND DOWN"

Those who are too rich for Medicaid have to pay for the nursing home themselves. Usually the rates are too high (averaging $50,000 a year nationally) for individuals to pay out of their own pockets for prolonged periods. They pay this amount until their money has been spent. This process is called the "spend down."

The economic equation that leads to placement of an elderly relative in a nursing home is much the same as that involved in placing children in day care—and is grimly sexist. If the woman can make more money working outside the home than the cost of day care, then the child is put in day care or the parent is placed in a nursing home. If the caregiver is a spouse, then he or she usually cannot work and will often struggle to keep the patient out of a nursing home to avoid the impoverishment created by the spend down. Fifty percent of all couples with one spouse in a nursing home become bankrupt.

The "spend down" creates some agonizing quandaries for families and even some qualms among state budget makers, and has given rise to a legal specialty of "poverty law." If the patient's assets must be dissipated before he or she becomes eligible for Medicaid, then what are the assets and what belongs to the family? In the past there were examples, and urban legends persist, of spouses getting divorced so that all their joint assets would not have to be spent. The more legislators have tried to prevent this, the more loopholes they have created for greedy heirs who want to preserve their inheritance while putting their parents in nursing homes on Medicaid.

The limits on what the patient or the family can keep are decided to a large extent by the federal government, but also in detail by the individual states. California allows the assets of a married couple to be divided as if a divorce had occurred when assessing eligibility for Medi-Cal. New York's 1989 Spousal Impoverishment Law allows the at-home spouse (as of 1998) to keep income up to $2,000 a month, and cash assets up to $80,000 besides a house and car.

LONG-TERM CARE INSURANCE

The Health Insurance Portability and Accountability Act of 1996 set uniform national standards for long-term care insurance and provided tax incentives for the purchase of plans that meet such standards. The New York State plan inaugurated in 1993 gives a tax break to those who insure themselves for at least three years of nursing home care at $100 a day (which is unrealistically low for New York) and promises that Medicaid will pick up the tab after three years (Mirabile, 1993).

It is doubtful whether long-term care insurance is a good buy outside of the element of direct government subsidy. Those who are rich enough can generally stay out of nursing homes and many people might be better off squirreling money away from the tax collector.

RESOURCE UTILIZATION GROUPS

The states have given Medicaid money to nursing homes according to a variety of formulas and methods, which previously varied considerably from state to state.

Originally, the most common method was based on the methods used to pay medieval armies and was known as "all you can steal." The nursing homes were asked how much they had spent on patient care each year and were then given that amount, plus a percentage over, as profit. New York used this system until it discovered that there was, to the state treasurer's surprise and grief, a tendency for nursing home proprietors to overstate what they had spent. Following this astounding revelation about human nature, several offenders were prosecuted amid great publicity, and various other methods were tried.

One method was known as "unto him that hath much, much shall be given." This was based on giving the nursing home the reimbursements as previously given, plus an allowance for inflation. This resulted in some nursing homes being paid $40 per day, and others $140 per day. The amount paid per patient simply depended on which nursing home they were in. In this way, New York State managed to spend, on 100,000 nursing home patients, $2.5 billion per year of state money. Thus, it was advantageous for nursing homes to retain patients who were not very ill. One excellent New York City nursing home proudly demonstrated its rehabilitative effort by staging a performance of *Guys and Dolls,* produced, sung, and acted by residents. The taxpayers of New York applauded the effort, but failed to understand why they should be paying $100 per day for the nursing care of the performers.

Such spectacular examples of successful rehabilitation were among the stimuli that led New York to change to RUGS (resource utilization groups). RUGS is an example of a kind of formula sometimes called "the sicker the better" or (more officially) "case-mix" reimbursement systems of the RUGS type. These systems are elaborate and time-consuming and do not really save money (Report by the Auditor General, State of California, 1987; Arling, Zimmerman, and Updike, 1989) but have now been federally mandated and are in effect in most states.

BALANCED BUDGET AMENDMENT AND PROSPECTIVE PAYMENT SYSTEM

BBA '97 (the Balanced Budget Amendment Act of 1997) has become almost as notorious in nursing home circles as OBRA '87. In particular it introduced the Prospective Payment System (PPS). The law was effective as of July 1, 1998, but the HCFA rules implementing the system allow for a phased-in approach with total implementation scheduled to be completed in four years (Beckwith, 1998; American Health Care Association, nd).

PPS makes the nursing homes pay for certain items, called "intrinsic" services, that were previously billed to Medicare Part B. Doctors' services provided by MDs are not affected by PPS and are designated as "extrinsic services." In addition to doctors' services, Part B of Medicare originally paid for many services in nursing homes that Medicaid does not cover, such as laboratory services. The nursing homes did not need to be concerned at all with the cost of anything that was covered by Part B of Medicare.

There may be some impact on medication use, and this could affect the use of the newer psychotropic drugs in nursing homes. In general, Medicare has never paid for medications except in certain limited circumstances. Generally speaking, nursing homes have had to pay for drugs, resulting in some pressure on doctors to prescribe cheaply, but exemptions have been made by many states, especially those where drug companies employ lobbyists, so that Medicaid pays for the expensive psychotropic drugs.

Another mental health issue may be payment for nonphysician mental health workers, such as social workers.

HEALTH MAINTENANCE ORGANIZATIONS

Health Maintenance Organizations (HMOs) grew rapidly from 1993 onward. This growth was not so much the result of any particular piece of federal legislation, as it was the result of failure to inaugurate various government health insurance plans that had been proposed as an answer to rapidly rising health care costs.

Because of the large role of Medicaid, which is already heavily regulated, and the complex interaction between Medicare and Medicaid, the impact of HMOs on nursing homes has been muted. If an HMO is covering Medicare but not Medicaid, then the HMO would be responsible for paying the doctors. In such a case, the HMO might find it more economical to have the patient in a nursing home than at home. If one controls for diagnoses and functional status, the costs to Medicare for nursing home residents are less than for those equally impaired living at home (Kane, 1999).

Outcry against HMOs has been particularly loud in psychiatry (and even louder among nonmedical providers of mental health care), mainly because of the limitations on hospitalization and on psychotherapy. These limitations have included the need for providers of these services to prove their necessity to a reviewer. The prescribing of psychotropic drugs and one-shot consultations have not been affected as much.

Medicare and Medicaid payments have been protected against the more rigorous exclusions. Sometimes patients who belong to an HMO that has a limited panel of providers whom it will pay are admitted to nursing homes. An exemption can usually be negotiated, but the process may be so time-consuming as not to be cost-effective for the practitioner. The result can be the patient goes without services and the HMO saves money.

THE BALLOON

In 1994, 1.6 million Americans lived in nursing homes, and this number is expected to triple by 2020 (Agronin, 1998). With the average nursing home costing $50,000 a year, something has to give sooner or later, particularly since the burden largely falls on Medicaid. The federal government pays $39 billion a year for nursing home care (*The New York Times,* 1999). Medicaid money that might help poor children is increasingly siphoned off into this gigantic middle-class subsidy.

Possibly this is disguised mental health expenditure. Only 1.5 percent of the Medicare budget goes to mental health services for the elderly (Bartels, 1998). This low proportion may represent the fact that the elderly mentally ill are receiving institutional care in the nursing homes.

For every inhabitant of New York over the age of eighty-five, the state spends $16,500 in nursing home Medicaid dollars. In other words, if Medicaid just handed $16,000 a year to every New Yorker over eighty-five, and did not subsidize any of them in nursing homes, it would be cheaper for the taxpayer. If the elderly are really competent to make their own financial decisions, then they might prefer to be given the money directly and to shop for their own best bargains in the health care marketplace (see Chapter 22).

Chapter 6

Anger at the Nursing Home

Anger at nursing homes is common. Books about nursing homes have such titles as *Tender Loving Greed* (Mendelson, 1975), *Death Without Dignity* (Long, 1987), and *Unloving Care* (Vladeck, 1980). Aggressive behavior by patients' families toward staff members is not uncommon. This may be purely verbal or staff may be slapped, punched, shoved, spat upon, or kicked. Daughters or stepdaughters of female patients are the most likely aggressors (Vinton, Mazza, and Kim, 1998).

COMPLAINTS

Most complaints about nursing homes are unsubstantiated (Mosca, 1999), although this may not mean they are completely groundless. Complaints come from patients, families, government inspectors, or the press. Complaints by patients are surprisingly uncommon. Patient complaints are often limited to very immediate grievances such as being deprived of a favorite chair, and are directed against other residents rather than the management.

Families complain, in order of frequency, about the laundry, the other patients, the food, and the quality of the medical and nursing care. Families will sometimes complain about lack of communication with the doctor, and this is more likely to happen in the nursing home than in the acute care general hospital. The problem is, paradoxically, less in large nursing homes in metropolitan areas, where one doctor sees many patients and makes a business of looking after nursing home patients. Although such doctors are strangers to the family, they will visit the nursing home frequently, if only to get paid.

In rural areas, where family doctors continue to serve patients they have known for a long time, doctors may only visit for the statutory minimum number of visits. This can be bewildering to the family when the patient was previously receiving daily hospital visits. They cannot understand why the doctor does not have up-to-date information. They are not accustomed to the nurse assuming the main responsibility. Consequently, the nurse may resent their reluctance to rely on him or her as the main source of information.

At the opposite extreme from the justified complaint is the situation in which the complaining family member is obviously mentally disturbed. Paranoia and schizophrenia are common illnesses affecting family members of nursing home patients. It is often helpful if a psychiatrist can directly field some of the telephone calls or interview the family member. When the patient has classic circular manic-depressive illness, then the likelihood exists that this same illness will affect a family member, as demonstrated in the following example:

> The daughter of a nursing home patient began making increasingly prolonged telephone calls expressing indignation at a psychiatrist's suggestion that her mother might be manic. She said that lithium should be avoided because she had been forced to take it herself and knew it caused radioactive fallout. She went on to express bizarre and grandiose delusions. Conversations had to be terminated by putting the telephone down, and she threatened to sue the psychiatrist. A few weeks later she was in his office suffering from a severe psychotic depression.

Dealing with Complaints

Every complaint may be justified and needs fair and vigorous investigation. The complainer must be assured that his or her concern is being addressed. Families are not aware of the health system's hierarchies and may complain to the wrong person. The medical director who receives a complaint about the marking of the laundry may feel that he or she is being bothered with trivialities and fail to investigate. It may seem that cupidity is involved when the family members emphasize the cost of a missing garment. One has to try to empathize with the fear that a loved relative is being clothed with institutional things from a common store.

Complaints by families about the other patients can understandably annoy the staff. A family that says, "Why is our mother with all these crazy people?" can be irritating, especially when the mother is as demented or disturbed as anyone else in the nursing home. Such complaints are more common when the demented are segregated. The family may feel their mother does not belong with the demented, or that she would be helped by being with more alert patients.

Dealing with such complaints must be a gradual process. Sometimes one can arrange to interview several patients together with the complaining family member present. The interview can demonstrate that the mother's memory and orientation are the same as that of the other patients.

The fact that dementia is the loved one's major illness may not be palatable or understandable for some families. They have been told that a physical illness is the official focus of medical attention. This can result in family members focusing on relatively small physical problems. Recently I had four telephone calls in two days about the progress of investigations into a slight anemia. The patient was in a nursing home and was deluded, hallucinating, and disoriented, with a progressive primary dementia. Anemia was, for this family, a socially acceptable illness that they could talk about and understand, and it gave them an acceptable reason for discussing the case with the doctor. Such families may be helped by being gradually introduced to the concept of dementia as a disease. They may need gradual suggestions that some of their relative's symptoms are caused by a disease of the brain. This can be done by introducing a discussion of memory and mood into discussions about physical symptoms, and making it clear that these are legitimate areas of medical and nursing concern. At a certain point contact with the Alzheimer's Association <www.alz.org> can be suggested, and the telephone number of the local chapter given.

When the family objects to a specific treatment method, such as blood transfusion or surgery, then this objection should be placed on record. Sometimes families will want a patient transferred to a hospital but will not want the specific treatments that would justify hospitalization in the eyes of the utilization review committee. (The many issues surrounding do not resuscitate (DNR) orders and the vigor with which medical treatment is pressed will be discussed in Chapter 20.)

NURSING HOME EXPOSÉS

News media and books from time to time expose dreadful conditions in nursing homes and the iniquities of those who work in them. The smell of urine and feces and the appearance of bedsores are described in vivid clichés.

Why is this? Perhaps nursing homes are, like funeral homes, a reminder of mortality. The residents are not the most popular members of a society that values youth and physical prowess. They are old and disabled. The families who put an aged relative in a nursing home wish they did not have to do it. They may feel frustrated and guilty. Even an eminent physician such as Talbott (1988) describes nursing homes as "deplorable places." What he probably means is that he does not enjoy being in them or feels he cannot do useful work in them.

Loebel and Rabitt (1988) point out that criticism of the quality of psychiatric care in nursing homes can have a negative effect on funding. Third-party payers (such as Medicaid) may be convinced that transinstitutionalization is taking place and that patients in nursing homes cannot possibly be getting adequate psychiatric care and, therefore, refuse to pay for any psychiatric care in nursing homes.

More serious is the effect on staff recruitment and on the morale of those already working in nursing homes. Those with access to the media should defend against irresponsible criticisms. There is a temptation for professionals to stay silent and keep a stiff upper lip. This is dignified but does not improve esprit de corps. Hotlines set up for complaints against nursing homes can be used as often as possible to say what a good job is being done and to press for diversion of funds from district attorneys' offices to patient care.

LITIGATION AGAINST NURSING HOMES

Five hundred million dollars a year, of which lawyers keep almost half, is made by suing nursing homes. In some states, such as Florida, if an elderly patient dies and the heirs can prove neglect, they can assuage their grief at their loss by collecting money from a lawsuit against the nursing home, even if the patient was on Medicaid. James Wilkes, of the Florida law firm Wilkes and McHugh, is a good example. Motivated, he says, by the trauma of having his grandmother die in a nursing home, Wilkes collected $35 million in nursing home legal settlements in 1998 (<www.wilkes-mchugh.com>).

Fear of Litigation

The fear of litigation, rather than its actuality, is an influence in nursing homes. Just as those without medical training have health superstitions, so those without legal training have legal superstitions. Many groundless fears of being sued are based on urban legends, and fear of being sued is sometimes given as a reason for patient care policies that cannot be otherwise rationally justified, such as the use of restraints previously discussed. Doubts and disagreements about intensity of care, transfer to hospital, or DNR orders are sometimes fueled by fear of litigation.

Government Inspectors

HCFA is the federal agency with authority to inspect nursing homes and enforce standards laid down by OBRA '87. HCFA delegates the authority to the states; of course, each state and local jurisdiction has its own rules governing everything from food preparation to pharmacy. All of these employ full-time inspectors of various kinds, often liable to descend unannounced at odd hours.

These government agencies are most likely to fault the home for not filling out forms properly. According to the American Health Care Association, the leading areas of deficiency have been comprehensive care plans, food, restraint use, and maintenance of an accident-free environment. According to HCFA the top cited areas were residents' rights, restraint use, and environment (*Provider*, 1991).

American Health Care Association

To some extent the nursing homes are defended by the American Health Care Association <www.ahca.org>. Although open to nonprofit nursing homes, the AHCA traditionally represents the much-maligned tax-paying nursing homes. It represents 12,000 homes, is headquartered in Washington, DC, and does a certain amount of lobbying.

MEASURING QUALITY OF CARE

Some nursing homes have an enviable reputation with the general public for being "good" nursing homes. Such a reputation will sometimes survive even well-publicized deficiencies found by inspectors, especially if the home is run by a religious or charitable organization. It is easy for a home to look "good" if it contains only the affluent and not very ill. The first target for exclusion by a home that wants to improve its public image is the patient with antisocial behaviors.

Measuring quality of care in any medical field is a complex matter with its own specialized terminology. Careful allowance has to be made for the fact that some institutions and doctors may be handling more difficult cases than others.

The commonly accepted terminology for assessing quality of care divides the assessment into three methods: structure, outcome, and process.

Structure

Structure refers to whether the buildings are new enough, the equipment good enough, and the staff numerous enough.

Outcome

Outcome is an important assessment but also the most difficult to measure. Outcome assesses whether the care makes patients better.

Process

Process measures are supposed to indicate whether the right things are being done. Most of the government instruments for assessing care quality, such as the MDS, measure process.

PART II:
THE PEOPLE

Chapter 7

The Families

Geriatrics rivals pediatrics in the extent of family involvement in decisions, but in some ways geriatric decisions are more difficult. Pediatrics usually involves just the parents. In geriatrics we have the complication of the extended family, and different family members may be involved to different extents. The complexity is further increased in the nursing home, because a complex organization, not just the individual practitioner, is at the receiving end.

The social, financial, and ethnic characteristics of nursing home patients will be further discussed in Chapter 9. These characteristics are reflected in their families. One result is that in many parts of the United States, especially urban areas, the families' backgrounds are different from those of the nursing home staff. This is a potential source of tension and communication difficulty.

THE ABSENT FAMILY

In many cases, the family of the nursing home patient is conspicuous by its absence. The childless, the unmarried, and the widowed are especially likely to be in nursing homes. However, this apparent absence can be deceptive.

Admissions often occur in the daytime on a weekday, and often at the time of admission there is a flurry of family activity, and extensive contact with relatives or friends. They visit frequently, and may want to know details of the food, the laundry, the dental care, and so forth. A phrase often heard at this time is, "You'll call us if there's any change." We as health professionals tend to forget the family said this, but the family does not forget.

After this initial flurry, many of the staff do not see much of the family for a while. The doctors, the social workers, the administrators, and the nursing staff on the day shift may rarely see them. Sometimes this is because the family members do not visit as much, but sometimes they may be visiting every night, without the day staff realizing it, or every weekend, without the office staff realizing it.

At this stage the presence of a concerned family may be forgotten, then the staff is taken by surprise when an indignant daughter wants to know why she was not called about her mother's fever or bedsore.

The Daughter from Ontario

The "daughter from Ontario" syndrome was described by Molloy and colleagues (1991). In the most extreme version of the syndrome, the patient is thought to have no family as none is on record. In other cases the information about family listed on the face sheet is misleading and the listed relatives are not the most concerned. Finding out who the concerned relative is may not be an easy matter and sometimes, even when the professionals or institution staff think they have done what is reasonable to consult with the family, the "daughter from Ontario" or "daughter from California" turns up, like the bad fairy at Sleeping Beauty's christening, indignant at not having been invited.

DISPUTES AMONG FAMILY MEMBERS

Disputes arise among family members. There may be requests that a particular relative or friend not be allowed to visit or take the patient out. The legality of such requests can be dubious. These situations are sometimes found in cases of second marriages. The children of the first marriage may be at odds with their stepparent. They may want to try to exclude him or her from decision making. Wherever the law gives one particular family member priority, the spouse is always chosen. The law still regards marriage as sacrosanct. Unmarried lovers have very little legal authority. When a rich old man becomes incompetent the resentful children can easily move in to exclude his mistress. It is important in such cases to place the patient's expressed wishes and degree of mental competence fully on record.

This is one of the reasons for failure of the plan in which one family member is the sole recipient of information, with the responsibility of passing it along to other family members. This sounds plausible in theory, but seldom works in practice except in the most straightforward of situations.

Wills and Testaments

Only lawyers can become completely familiar with the nuances of testamentary capacity, powers of attorney, and competence to enter into contracts in every state. (Living wills are discussed in Chapter 20.) It is important to have at least some facts on the chart about the patient's mental state. It is embarrassing to go to court as a witness about a million dollar estate and give testimony based on a record of less than a half-page about the patient's mental status. The judges do not demand much. Can the patient add and subtract? Does the patient know how much money he or she has?

THE DIFFICULT FAMILY

Certain families are labeled by the staff as difficult. (However, not all of the staff label the same families.) Families who complain a lot about nursing homes are not always bad people. In fact, the contrary may be true. These are the very families who care deeply about every aspect of the care of their relative and cannot tolerate the thought of the loved one suffering discomfort. I have often followed patients in my office or their homes who were the object of selfless devotion by kind and caring families, who expressed great appreciation of my medical care. Then, when they finally gave up and the patient was admitted to a nursing home, with me having told the staff what a nice family this was, I find the family giving hell to the nursing home staff. The nurses want to know how I could ever have thought these querulous nuisances were nice.

The Overburdened Family

The burden of caring for a disabled relative at home is severe and admission to a nursing home does not always end the burden. Abusive, able-bodied, demented men are sometimes kept at home because it is difficult to convince nursing homes to take them, but their wives face criticism if they do finally institutionalize them (Bédard et al., 1999). Some families, dependent on a double income, make frantic attempts to keep up with obligations by frequent visiting and feel caught in a rat race.

Such families have to cope with feeling that it is for the sake of the mortgage on the house in the suburbs, or the child's college tuition, that Grandma was put in a home. Those who aspire to such ideas are often educated people with strong consciences. From these families we hear such phrases as, "We cannot manage her at home because we both work," or, more usually, "We both must work."

In one family I know, the husband and wife have both sets of parents in nursing homes. They spend all their free time visiting four nursing homes, to the neglect of the children whose Ivy League education they are paying for. They are hard-working, law-abiding taxpayers, with well-behaved children who are excellent students. However, they feel guilty knowing that the cost to the taxpayer of looking after their parents is more than that of supporting four welfare mothers with twelve children.

Psychiatric Illness in the Family

Stress and mental illness cannot be equated; and although stressed caregivers may describe themselves as anxious or depressed, they seldom become mentally ill in the sense of needing psychiatric treatment (Eagles et al., 1987). Silliman and colleagues (1986) in North Carolina compared the families who cared for stroke victims at home with those who had them institutionalized and found a lack of significant difference. The home caregivers suffered from loss of time for themselves and from financial burdens, but those with institutionalized family members also suffered from these. It is probably more emotionally taxing to deal with disability in a spouse than in a parent (Carnwath and Johnson, 1987).

Apart from depression, other psychiatric illness within the family can become the concern of the nursing home. This sometimes associates with the phenomenon of two generations of aging. Nursing home residents are often in their nineties, and can have children who are in their sixties and beginning to suffer age-related infirmities themselves. When the most involved relative is a spouse, one of the most common illnesses the nursing home has to deal with is dementia. Nursing home staff may be the first to become aware of the spouse's dementia and may need to bring it to the attention of other family members or social agencies. It may sometimes have been a toss-up which one of a couple was to be institutionalized.

With the most difficult families, mutual support for the staff becomes especially important. A staff meeting, scheduled to get staff from different shifts and disciplines together can help everyone ventilate their frustrations and formulate an approach. The staff will tend to interpret family anger as guilt, and I do not quarrel with this diagnosis when I am talking to them. It is often useful to discuss the concepts mentioned in this chapter with the staff. At such meetings it may emerge that the problem is not the entire family, but one or two members. Identifying a reasonable and responsible family member can be most useful.

The drastic remedy of dismissing the patient is sometimes invoked but is seldom necessary and, indeed, may fail to alleviate the situation. It may not be possible to discharge the patient and the complaints may continue after the patient has gone.

Contact between patients' families for mutual support can sound threatening to nursing home staff, but can be constructive. A group of this kind can be organized informally and may provide a certain amount of group therapy. Organizing a formal support group is difficult work, seldom reimbursed by insurance, but has rewards in other areas. Where one nursing home serves a wide area, the nursing home may be a suitable venue for meetings of the local Alzheimer's Disease Association.

Although there are no good statistical studies, my experience has been that the prognosis of the difficult family is surprisingly good. Most of them seem to settle down eventually, or the staff finds ways of dealing with them.

Chapter 8

The Staff

Most workers in nursing homes are in entry-level positions, mainly as nurse assistants, but also as kitchen workers or cleaners (Watson, 1991). Nursing facilities, as opposed to board and care homes and assisted living facilities, are required to provide care by registered nurses, and to employ a medical director and several other mandated professionals. Some of these other mandated professionals in the nursing home have a crucial role in mental health care. Food and fluid refusal, or weight loss due to depression, involve the dietician. The dietetic service supervisor is commonly a registered dietician (RD) licensed by the Commission on Dietetic Registration, but may have lesser qualifications if an RD provides consultation and supervision.

Federal law requires that every nursing facility have "an ongoing program of activities," which must be directed by a qualified therapeutic recreation specialist or occupational therapist. These professionals are the backbone of the programs that ensure that patients do not spend their days parked in front of a television set. They may direct such therapies as Reality Orientation and Remotivation.

OWNERS AND ADMINISTRATORS

In some small nursing homes, especially outside New York, Florida, and California, the administrator may be the owner; but this is unusual in the larger nursing homes in the larger states and is becoming rarer. Such owner-administrators may only have the minimum number of hours of training mandated by the state for nursing home administrators.

Most administrators are male and have at least a bachelor's degree with further training in geriatrics; administrators often have a master's degree in administration or public health. The administrator gets a bigger salary than any other employee, including the Director of Nursing Services (DNS), who is the top nurse. The administrator is appointed by the owners and is ultimately responsible for hiring and firing the rest of the staff, including the Medical Director and the DNS. One justification for the large income is that the administrator is largely responsible for the financial end of things. When nursing homes lose money, the administrators lose their jobs.

NURSE ASSISTANTS

Most nursing home employees are classified as "nurse assistants," commonly called "aides," and they deliver most of the care (DeRuvo-Keegan, 1992). Until OBRA there was no federal standard for training aides. Nursing homes could hire anyone who walked in, regardless of education or training, and the individual could start work immediately as a nursing aide. Many of those hired in this way are doing excellent jobs. Regulations now specify that nursing aides must have some course of training, although the value of such training is unproven (Goldman and Woog, 1975), and they must take an examination that includes evidence of proficiency in the English language.

In rural areas the nursing aides may come from the same milieu as the patients, but in city and suburban areas they will come from different milieus, usually reflecting the cheapest and most willing workers (Tellis-Nayak and Tellis-Nayak, 1989). Some of the younger ones want to explore a health care job, and may later go on to become LPNs, RNs, MDs, or investigative journalists exposing the inadequacies of nursing home care. In the inner cities, the aides are mostly African Americans. In the suburbs, these are joined by Asian and other immigrants who are relatively new in the United States and cannot get any other job. These immigrants are often intelligent and hardworking. They may include persons of high education whose professional skills are not marketable in the United States. Nursing aide work is relatively unpopular among Hispanics, however.

Ethnicity and ethnic tensions remain important factors in nursing homes, especially in areas such as New York City, where most of the elderly were born outside the United States (Gurland et al., 1983) and where some homes have residents who belong to predominantly one ethnic group (Flint, 1982). Many of the elderly with mild dementia will display crude racial prejudices. They may shout racial epithets at aides and refuse to be cared for by aides who are not white.

Cultural differences cause an emotional strain on the aides in other ways as well. To make one's living in a foreign country is difficult enough without doing it in a nursing home. Many of them live in two isolated worlds. They come from a background that is isolated from the mainstream of American life, and then they go to work in a milieu which is also isolated from the mainstream.

The American born aides may feel relatively underpaid and that they are there to enable the families of their patients to go off and earn bigger salaries. Many of the female aides have small children and work out of sheer economic necessity.

A less obvious but very strong grievance of the aides is the lack of any kind of praise or positive feedback for their work. The importance of this is emphasized in several studies (Caudill and Patrick, 1989). It is not, therefore, surprising that aides in nursing homes have very high rates of absenteeism. Their job turnover averages 40 percent (Waxman, Carner, and Berkenstock, 1984).

THE NURSES

Nursing homes, by definition, are places in which nursing is practiced. The most precious commodity in the nursing home is the time of the skilled nurse. At least one RN must be on duty eight hours a day, and at least one LPN twenty-four hours a day. The RN, performing hands-on bedside duties, has become an endangered species in the United States, although attempts to abolish the actual word nurse, because of its sexist and hierarchal connotations, have failed.

Licensed Practical Nurses

At one time it was expected that Licensed Practical Nurses (LPNs, called Licensed Vocational Nurses in California and Texas) would replace RNs in hospitals, but hospitals have preferred to train technicians to perform hands-on technical procedures, and an increasing proportion (at present 25 percent) of the 700,000 U.S. LPNs work in nursing homes. LPNs tend to like nursing home work because of the autonomy and responsibility they are given (Brannon et al., 1988), although they are poorly paid.

Motivations of Nursing Home Nurses

Why do nurses choose to work in nursing homes? First, let it be said that there are those who are dedicated to the good that they can do and who find special satisfaction in serving the very helpless and in rehabilitating long-term patients.

There are some other positive attractions. The nursing home is not required to have a registered nurse on all shifts, therefore, the registered nurse can be offered the possibility of a job limited to day shifts. Because there are more nursing homes than hospitals, more job flexibility is available, including the opportunity to find a job closer to home. These are advantages that appeal mainly to female nurses who are married and have children at home, and possibly why it is unusual to find a male RN in a nursing home.

Also, the nursing home nurse provides more autonomy and responsibility. The hospital is very hierarchical; doctors and administrators and supervisors are everywhere. In the nursing home, the registered nurses feel more in charge. Deckard, Hicks, and Rowntree (1986) found that registered nurses in nursing homes were fairly comfortable with their lot and appreciated the greater autonomy and responsibility of nursing home work although they were discontented that additional responsibility was not reflected in increased salaries. Cohen-Mansfield (1989) also found nursing staff held generally positive attitudes toward their work.

Psychological Problems of Nurses

Nurses who find themselves working in a nursing home because they must, and who have been used to acute care general hospitals, may be frightened by the lonely responsibility. Some nurses suffer from anxiety, centered around the fear of harming a patient. This pervasive fear commonly causes nurses to leave the profession.

These fears do not favor the nursing home patient. A fear of some technical error, such as a drug overdose, can lead, for example, to insistence on bed rest, because this seems safer than mobilization.

Good geriatric practice can conflict with the nurse's previous medical practice in the acute care general hospital. This arouses anxiety and can lead to loss of nursing staff unless indoctrination and education in geriatrics can be provided.

The behavior of doctors is a major complaint of nurses. Sometimes when nurses are required by regulations to telephone doctors, the doctors are unpleasant (Cadogan et al., 1999).

Nurse Practitioners and Physician Assistants

Some evidence suggests that use of primary care teams involving nurse practitioners provides optimal care in nursing homes, although measures of this, such as frequency of transfer to emergency rooms, are of dubious validity (Boult, 1999).

The nurse practitioner (NP) differs from the physician assistant (PA) in usually having first qualified as an RN. NPs are more likely to be female, to function as a primary care practitioner, and to be independent of MDs. The PA tends to work in a high technology, specialized field under closer MD supervision. Nurse practitioners who work in nursing homes spend more time with the patients than MDs (Gold, 1999), usually due to economic reasons. MDs find that nursing home work is less lucrative. Perhaps MDs can skimp on paperwork and bend rules and cut corners without affecting real quality of care. NPs are usually paid by Part B of Medicare and Medicaid, but arrangements for this can be complicated by state requirements about MD supervision.

THE DOCTORS

Physicians who work in nursing homes are frequent targets of criticism (Turnbull, 1989). It is claimed that they are seldom involved in staff training, perfunctory in their visits, unfamiliar with regulatory standards, and prescribe drugs without seeing or knowing anything about the patients.

Such criticisms do not add to the attractiveness of nursing home work for doctors. The typical doctor visits the nursing home with reluctance, if at all. Young internists starting out in practice may take on a few nursing home patients, but give these up when they get busy.

They find demented elderly patients with multiple ailments frustrating. They have not been trained in the technique of examining or estimating the functional capacity of these patients. The old-line general practitioner may follow patients into the nursing home. Such continuity of primary care might be expected to be beneficial, but Susman, Zervanos, and Byerly (1989) were not able to demonstrate any improvement in outcome resulting from continuity of care between hospital and nursing home by a primary care physician.

Although the public may have little sympathy for any doctor who complains about being underpaid, the present payment system provides little financial incentive for the doctor to visit the nursing home, especially if he or she is treating only one or two patients. Such a visit may earn a tenth of the money but take the same amount of time as a technical procedure such as a colonoscopy, which can be done in the office. If called about a patient who is seriously ill, it is more financially feasible for the doctor to order the patient sent to the hospital.

The doctor's primary source of income from nursing home patients is Medicare. Typically, Medicare will only pay for one visit per patient per month. An additional visit may be paid for if it can be justified as medically necessary. Medicare will quite often refuse to pay for services in nursing homes that must be provided by a doctor. On some occasions a visit to pronounce death has been disallowed, with a notice of denial sent to the deceased patient stating, "This many visits not necessary for your condition." Avorn (1998) has pointed out that the elderly in nursing homes often get less attention (but more medication) from their doctors than do their free-living counterparts. This paradox arises because their contact with the doctor is limited to visits at the time of the doctor's (or Medicare's) choice, or is mediated, and thus to some extent censored, by nursing staff.

In the early days of Medicare notorious examples of "gang visits" abounded. The doctor would visit a nursing home containing 100 or more patients, not leave the administrator's office, yet charge for having seen all the patients. Such abuses led Medicare to insist on documentation of visits to each patient, which led in turn to more of the dreaded paperwork.

Some altruistic and dedicated doctors with an interest in geriatrics may rise above these mere monetary considerations, and some may say such considerations do not matter; but the invisible hand of the marketplace is always at work advising the doctor not to spend too much time in the nursing home. The staff tends to perceive the doctor as reluctant to visit and anxious to leave. Such anxious doctors may remain at the nursing station rather than examine patients, may be unaware of whether the patient can walk or stand or control the bladder or bowels, and may prescribe symptomatically, giving Lomotil to those with diarrhea and diuretics to those with swollen feet.

The Medical Director

The medical director is not the grand figure that the title suggests, and the status of the position has fallen from its original intention. The original legislation that required each nursing home to employ a physician as medical director was passed in 1972 as a result of earlier nursing home scandals. The idea then was that putting a doctor in charge would ensure reform. In theory, medical directors were responsible for organizing the medical staff and ensuring that they did their work properly, but this may not have been much of a reality in the smaller homes. They were supposed to advise the administrator and DNS about medical matters and sit on committees. The appointed medical directors were typically recruited from the ranks of older, local, male family doctors of the generation who were not certified in any specialty (rather than the newer breed with family practice certification). They spent less than five hours a week at the facility, most of which was spent visiting their own patients (Birkett, 1980).

The role of medical director as the guardian of quality care has now been assumed by the regulatory agencies. Speculation about eliminating the requirement arose with OBRA '87, but it was retained and reinforced. In spite of this, the role has declined rather than increased. Many medical directors are discontented with the extent of their control over nursing home policies (Elon, 1993). In fact, many nursing homes apparently get by without any paid medical director at all (McCarthy, Banaszak-Hall, and Fries, 1999). They presumably comply with the letter of the law by designating a local doctor as medical director. If paid at all, the post of medical director is poorly reimbursed by medical standards and is often held by a semiretired doctor (Cefalu, 1998).

Efforts to improve this situation are being made by the American Medical Directors Association, which has instituted a certifying examination for medical directors. In some ways the formation of such groups as the American Medical Directors Association parallels that of the Association of Superintendents of Asylums for the Insane which evolved into the American Psychiatric Association.

An active medical director with a keen interest in geriatrics and chronic care can do a great deal to improve the morale and atmosphere of a small nursing home. However, the most active medical directors are typically found in large nursing homes with teaching hospital affiliations. In some of the major metropolitan areas, the medical director is a full-time, salaried, board-certified physician. In homes affiliated with medical schools, the medical director is more likely to be certified by the American Medical Directors Association and/or in internal medicine by the American Board of Medical Specialties, in some cases with subspecialty certification in geriatrics.

Geriatricians

An obstacle to the development of a separate specialty of geriatrics has been a certain stigmatization and association with rationing of care. The affluent and nondemented elderly prefer to use "organ-based" specialists (Banerjee, 1998). In spite of this, a reading of a few issues of *Gerontologist* or the *Journal of the American Geriatrics Society* will reveal that there is a lively and developing specialty of geriatrics. Many brilliant young doctors have been intrigued by the biology of aging and the quest for immortality. The mysteries of Alzheimer's disease and dementia are attracting some of medicine's keenest minds. Some of these are in pure research in the laboratory, but some also become involved in clinical work. Highly motivated internists may welcome the opportunity to observe the classical physical signs of disease in a chronic care situation. If one wants to teach physical signs to medical students, the nursing home is a good place to find cases.

Good doctors are attracted to large nursing homes that are closely affiliated with equally large teaching hospitals. Such nursing homes are common in large metropolitan centers and are able to attract good doctors with an interest in research in geriatrics. A drawback is that such nursing homes lose out in the competition for nursing staff. They have to compete with the acute care general hospitals for nurses but have lost the features that attract nurses to nursing homes.

Psychiatrists

Psychiatrists, like most other doctors, are reluctant to treat the elderly. Their typical patients range between twenty and sixty years old and only 0.6 percent of their patients are seen in nursing homes (NDTI Specialty Profile, 1998). The American Psychiatric Association has 42,000 members but the American Association for Geriatric Psychiatry has only 2,000 members. Smaller and more rural nursing homes do not often have available psychiatric consultants (Reichman et al., 1998). Probably more psychiatrists see the younger patients in the adult homes and board and care homes, but statistics are scarce.

Medicare payments discourage psychiatric treatment, especially psychotherapy. At one time all psychiatric services were paid for at a lower rate, called "level Z," and often not paid for at all. The decision that a service was psychiatric hinged on the diagnosis. If the stated diagnosis was, for example, depression, then payment for seeing the patient was cut in half. This has largely been abolished, although it still applies to long-term psychotherapy given without prescribing medication.

Reimbursement to psychiatrists is only possible, unless the home is unusually affluent, for extrinsic services. Extrinsic services involve an outside professional who practices independently. Intrinsic services are part and parcel of nursing home care. Providing intrinsic services enables psychiatrists to perform such functions as talking to staff and attending team meetings to formulate care plans, but intrinsic services are subject to the financial limitations of BBA and PPS (see Chapter 5).

We return to the fact that the present system involves trying to treat severely ill psychiatric patients in a setting that is officially nonpsychiatric. Psychiatric management of severely ill mental patients in an institution necessitates control of the environment and a close relationship with the treatment team.

In the nursing home the patient is allocated a primary care physician on the same basis as in the acute care general hospital. (The situation is different in the adult homes and board and care homes, where there is no assigned doctor and patients choose their physicians on the same basis as do the noninstitutionalized.) In the old state mental hospital system the psychiatrist filled this role, but the generation of psychiatrists with the expertise and motivation for this has largely vanished. Psychiatrists today base their medical identity on expertise in psychopharmacology rather than in neurology and general medicine. A factor that may cause them to regret their loss of skills is that newer psychotropic drugs are so free of side effects and so easy to use that the need for a psychiatrist to prescribe them is lessening.

In general, anyone with a single diagnosed disease will get better treatment from a doctor who specializes in that disease. This has been shown in studies of several different illnesses. However, elderly nursing home patients seldom have the good judgment to confine themselves to a single illness.

Psychiatric Consultations

The kinds of mental disorders commonly found in nursing home surveys are not typically those that lead to nursing home consultations by psychiatrists. Withdrawn and apathetic types of depression or schizophrenia are unlikely to be causes for requesting consultation. If these illnesses result in consultation request it is because of a disturbed behavior, such as food refusal, violence, or suicide attempt.

Although dementia is the most prevalent condition found in the surveys, it is very seldom given as the reason for the consultation. Even when the patient is demented, a psychiatrist will not be brought in to help look for the cause of the dementia, but for some additional behavior problem. This may occur because under OBRA rules, the mentally disordered can only be placed in nursing homes if they are demented, and the diagnosis of dementia should have been made and investigated and substantiated before the patient came in. Nevertheless, the consultant should always place on record some quantified assessment of the degree of memory and cognitive impairment. As in general hospital liaison psychiatry, the causes of acute confusional state may need to be reviewed, with particular reference to the possibility of multiple medication.

Nursing home staff often want the psychiatrist to recommend medications and give a diagnosis rather than get involved in general psychosocial management (Reichman et al., 1998). Some consultation requests seem to be requests for sedation, or ordered so as to document the existence of mental disorder to justify medication in accordance with OBRA requirements. As a result, recommendations for treatments other than medication are ignored, and the medication recommendation alone is followed. Sometimes it is best to defer any recommendation of medication until other methods have been tried and to ask for a report on the efficacy of these measures before giving a recommendation for medication. If a psychotropic drug is recommended, the family must be informed about the drug and its side effects.

In establishing rapport with the nursing staff, the psychiatrist should determine which shift is most disturbed by the patient's behavior. The night shift may be upset because a patient does not stay in bed at night and insists on getting up and walking around, but the day shift may think they have a nice quiet patient. Shifts commonly change at 3 p.m., and there are pros and cons to arriving at this time. The day shift may be in a hurry to finish up their paperwork and hand over to the next shift. However, this is often a good time to start a dialogue between the shifts. When the day shift finishes their work they are sometimes in clined to hang around to talk about the patient at their leisure.

Requests from administrators, medical directors, or directors of nursing services often arise from an administrative problem, such as placement, legal capacity, or the need to satisfy some bureaucratic state requirement. The request may require the completion of a particular form or a specific kind of report. The psychiatrist should make sure which form is needed before starting the report. Sometimes the reason for the referral involves placement. Where does the patient belong in the spectrum of available care? *Available* is the key word here. The consultant who believes that the patient belongs on an inpatient psychiatric service will often find this difficult to arrange. Patients with concomitant physical conditions are unacceptable in many psychiatric units. State-funded facilities will often simply refuse to accept patients under the guise of keeping the patient "in the community." The private practitioner must then get on the telephone to explain that, whatever the virtues of the home, it is an institution, and not the best one for that particular patient at that particular time.

In many cases, the psychiatrist consults as representative of a publicly funded agency, such as Mobile Geriatric Teams. In such cases he or she will also have to ascertain, preferably unequivocally and in writing, the policies of the employing state agency. If the referral is from the nursing home for the purpose of hospitalization, then the psychiatrist sent by a state agency with a policy of avoiding hospitalization may be caught in a cleft stick.

When the request comes from the patient's family, this is often an indication that the patient is in actual subjective distress from depression or anxiety. Depressed patients who have previously responded well to organic treatments will sometimes be referred from this familial source. The patient becomes withdrawn and inactive, and while the nursing home staff do not notice much wrong, the family remembers that last time their loved one was like this he or she responded well to electric shock treatment. Sometimes families want individual psychotherapy on a regular basis, and it may be difficult to explain to them that this cannot realistically be given in a nursing home. Pleading exigencies of money and time may lead the families to feel that their relative is being denied a necessary treatment because of lack of money. A reasonable response to this may be to offer the treatment in a private office if the family is willing to transport the patient.

A visiting psychiatrist may find that he or she is repeatedly called upon concerning the same patient, and it becomes evident that the patient is primarily a psychiatric case. Repeated visits by a psychiatrist to the same patient may not be reimbursed.

Probably the best solution in cases in which the primary diagnosis is psychiatric is for the psychiatrist to become the primary care physician. This is particularly apposite in those cases where there is no major medical problem below the neck. The main advantage to the patient with a primary care physician with psychiatric expertise is not merely in having psychological needs attended to, but in reduction of physical morbidity and of mortality. This reduction is partly due to avoidance of multiple medications, and to more accurate recognition of physical symptoms based on depression. The psychiatrically trained physician tends to use psychotropic medication more appropriately, and thus cause less sedation and adverse drug effects.

A disadvantage is that some psychiatrists, especially those trained in American teaching hospitals, feel they lack training and experience in primary care medicine. The older generation is more comfortable with this role, especially those trained in state hospitals or those (often foreign medical graduates) who had extensive training in other fields before specializing in psychiatry. Distrust of the psychiatrist as primary care physician may come from the nursing staff or family. New fellowship training programs in geriatric psychiatry may turn out psychiatrists who are competent general physicians and geriatricians.

The psychiatrist who visits the nursing home on a private pay, fee-for-service basis to do a one-shot consultation has limited influence. Various ways around this have been tried. In some nursing homes, the psychiatrist calls on a regular basis and also sits with the staff and discusses the psychiatric aspects of current cases. This is desirable, but raises the question of who pays the psychiatrist.

Tourigny-Rivard and Drury (1987) describe a system of monthly visits to a nursing home by a psychiatrist, with specific patients being seen in consultation and an in-service being provided for staff at the same session. By their account, based on a single nursing home, this worked well, and they were able to document improvements in staff self-confidence and morale, and a reduction in psychiatric emergencies, although measurable patient improvement was not noticed.

Psychotherapy

What about the provision of nonmedication types of treatment? Does psychotherapy in its classical sense, the prolonged one-on-one conversation, have a place in the nursing home? Doubt has been cast on this, and it has even been suggested that such services may be excessive and unjustified (American Psychiatric Association, 1998). If PASARR screening shows that the nursing home patient needs specialized mental health services, and the nursing home responds by providing fifty-minute sessions with a mental health professional once a week to a demented patient, then have the needed services been provided? What is to prevent a mental health professional from providing superfluous and unneeded services? Provision of "extrinsic" services often provokes such suspicions.

Probably the psychosocial aspects of treatment are best provided as part of "intrinsic" rather than "extrinsic" mental health services (see BBS). This leaves the problem of getting professional mental health input into the intrinsic serves. The traditional type of written consultation, as we have seen, does not always achieve this. Attendance at multidisciplinary care plan meetings where individual patients are discussed is often more productive, but psychiatrists in private practice can normally only get paid for direct patient care.

"Group therapy" for the elderly demented is especially likely to be suspected of not being a legitimate therapeutic activity (Bartels, 1998; Bartels and Colenda, 1998). There has been a fear that such therapy might be a euphemism for "gang visits" and a corresponding difficulty in reimbursement, even to the point of Medicare fraud accusations. It is always difficult to evaluate effectiveness in nursing homes because of the special difficulty in arranging control groups. Many of the papers are descriptive and anecdotal (e.g., Saul, 1974).

Moses (1982) describes a program of group therapy in nursing homes conducted by nonprofessionals who were given 120 hours of training. No untreated patient control group is mentioned. There was initial enthusiasm but the project was dropped. The group leaders apparently came from within the staff of the nursing home, and this was a factor in dropping the project. The group leaders felt pressured for time, and felt that they were under an obligation to increase their workload. There are two lessons to be drawn from the Moses study. The first is that anything done for the purpose of helping the patient's mental condition can arouse staff enthusiasm. The second is the value of the visiting mental health professional. The staff feel that any treatment is better than none. Compared with drugs, consultations, or in-service instruction, a professionally led group makes the staff feel that, at a specific place and a specific time, the patient is getting treatment.

It seems likely that this factor of increased staff morale within the home is greater if the groups are conducted by someone with special training who comes in from the outside. If existing staff members are used they may find the work regarded as an addition to their other duties, rather than a substitute for them. They will be recruited into other activities that the home regards as more essential when the home is short of staff. The other activities regarded as more essential will be hands-on caregiving or technical nursing tasks.

OTHER MENTAL HEALTH PROFESSIONALS

Social Workers

A facility with more than 120 beds must employ a full-time qualified social worker, defined in the federal regulations as an individual with either a bachelor's degree in social work or two years of supervised social work experience in a health care setting. The social worker in a nursing home usually has a social work degree (MSW or BSW) or a bachelor's degree that has included social work plus a year of experience, and has obtained certification by the state or the Academy of Social Workers (ACSW). Social workers with lesser qualifications must be supervised by a social services consultant.

The social worker will often be the staff's strongest advocate for the residents' psychosocial welfare, and the person who is most knowledgeable about their backgrounds outside the home. The social worker is often burdened with chores that no one else wants to do, such as telephoning, writing, or billing. Nursing home work is, therefore, not very popular among social workers, who tend to think of nursing homes as derelict backwaters.

The psychosocial history mandated by law is mostly written out by the social worker and usually gives better information about the patient's mental condition than any other piece of paper in the chart.

Psychiatric Nurses

Psychiatric nurses may come to the nursing home as members of outside governmental agencies, such as the Mobile Geriatric Teams. More and more, they work on a part-time basis in nursing homes, and thus are perceived as employees rather than consultants, and as being there to complete the required government documentation. This can be seen as pure paperwork. The papers are filled out; the nurse departs; the papers are filed away. The psychiatric nurses must be assertive to make an impact on patient care; but, if they are female, this assertiveness is resented. It is easier, in the short run, to lapse into a passive and subordinate role. A great deal of sophistication about health care hierarchies, as well as about geriatric psychiatry, is called for. The psychiatric nurse should write reports on a consultation sheet, rather than in the nursing notes, and have them typed.

Psychologists

Regrettably, psychologists play a small part in the nursing home. For example, many aspects of the evaluation of communication disorders and dementia can be best elucidated by a neuropsychologist. It is difficult to obtain third-party reimbursement for psychological services in the nursing home. Occasionally, reports by a psychologist are legally mandated, especially when the mentally retarded are involved, and the patient has to pay out of his or her Supplemental Security Income spending allowance.

Many of the staff issues in nursing homes are the same as those in other organizations, such as hospitals, but these issues are of greater significance in the nursing home than in the general hospital because there is less equipment around to get in the way (Brannon et al., 1988). The final product of the nursing home is a beneficial result produced for people by people.

Chapter 9

The Patients

The typical nursing home resident is an eighty-five-year-old child-less white widow in a Midwestern state. She is moderately demented and takes several medications, including Haldol (haloperidol), a diuretic, a laxative, and a medication for pain. She looked after her husband until he died, then a year or two later she was put in the home. She was once moderately prosperous but is now an impoverished Medicaid recipient. She is unsteady on her feet and is strapped to a chair much of the time. She has been in the nursing home for two years, never leaves it, and will die there. If she once lived by herself in a house that she owned, the house was probably sold to pay for her nursing home care. Part of the reason she has to stay in the nursing home is that she no longer has a home to go to (Berthold, Landahl, and Svanborg, 1988).

In what ways does she differ from the rest of us? The differences are only partly due to her age and medical condition. It is possible to be quite old or quite ill and stay out of a nursing home. The differences may be classified as age, sex, socioeconomic status, and psychiatric and medical conditions.

AGE

Simply being very old is one reason for being in a nursing home. Every twentieth American over sixty-five years of age is in a nursing home (Aging Health Policy Center, 1986), and most centenarians are institutionalized. Board and care homes occupied by former state hospital patients contain a relatively young group, although even here the elderly predominate.

Young Nursing Home Residents

Nearly 20 percent of nursing home bed days are accounted for by those under sixty-five. This youngest group is the most likely to be truly medically ill. The young are more likely to be in nursing homes because of the severity of their illnesses rather than socioeconomic causes. Young people who are socially isolated and destitute end up in the street rather than the nursing home. In the board and care homes the most common illness among the young is schizophrenia, often combined with varying degrees of drug and alcohol abuse.

The young in the nursing homes, apart from the mentally retarded, have usually suffered a devastating illness or (very commonly) injury, and a large part of the psychology of dealing with them is that of dealing with the victims of such conditions. It is rare to find a young person in a nursing home who does not have a condition affecting the nervous system. These youngsters are demoralized by their illness and by being in a nursing home, but also suffer mental changes from the organic effects of their illness on the brain.

SEX

Most nursing home residents are women and most of them are widowed. The female preponderance is obviously due in part to women living longer than men, although men actually live as long as women in terms of healthy functioning lives. The extra years that are granted to women are often years of illness and dementia. A large number of social factors could be at work. It is possible that men are kept out of nursing homes because they are looked after by their wives when they get sick. However, sometimes when a husband dies, we find that he was being leaned on as well as leaning. Many husbands compensate for their wives' dementia, and the severity of the woman's dementia becomes apparent only in widowhood. Men do not survive in nursing homes as long as women (Breuer et al., 1998).

Are there too many women in nursing homes compared with men? Some reallocation might be fair. The burden of Alzheimer's disease in men on wives is greater than that of Alzheimer's disease in women on men for several reasons (Bédard et al., 1999). Abusive, able-bodied, demented men are sometimes kept at home because nursing homes will not take them. Women are pressured to take care of their husbands and face criticism if they do not.

SOCIOECONOMIC STATUS

The pretense that patients are put in nursing homes because of medical conditions becomes more obvious when we look at geographic variation and social and economic profiles. The typical patient's background and ethnic affiliations are middle class. The very rich do not enter nursing homes. The very poor also keep out. This may be because Grandma's Social Security check is an important part of the household income, and she owns the house or has the lease on the rent-controlled apartment where the family lives.

The part of the country in which she lives will strongly affect her chances of being in a nursing home. In Nebraska, Montana, Oklahoma, and Kansas almost every tenth person over sixty-five years of age is in a nursing home; this is more than three times the number of persons in nursing homes in West Virginia, Florida, or the District of Columbia. More than one percent of the population of North and South Dakota and of Iowa were living in nursing homes in 1990, but Midwestern states also had the highest proportions of elderly living alone (U.S. Bureau of the Census, 1993).

Blacks and Hispanics are underrepresented in nursing homes as patients (Cohen, Hyland, and Magai, 1998) although not as staff. This underrepresentation may be because African Americans do not live as long as individuals of European ancestry. Weissert and Cready (1988) adduced evidence suggesting that discrimination might also be a factor. Hispanics also are underrepresented in nursing homes because of the young composition of this ethnic group. Some ethnic and religious groups may do a better job of keeping their aged relatives home with the family.

African-American and Hispanic nursing home residents are generally more cognitively and functionally impaired than white non-Hispanic residents (Chiodo et al., 1994) and less likely to receive a diagnosis of depression (Cohen, Hyland, and Magai, 1998).

PSYCHIATRIC AND MEDICAL CONDITIONS

If we exclude medical consequences of dementia, and look for a nondemented patient who is in a nursing home purely because of a medical illness, such a person is difficult to find, in spite of the medical illnesses recorded on the face sheets as the reasons for admission. This is not to say that none of them are medically ill. Many victims of severe medical illness are in the nursing homes, but just as many are not. Medical severity and chronicity do not in and of themselves lead to nursing home placement. Most young quadriplegics, for example, stay home. So far, then, the differences between nursing home patients and the rest of us relate to social, rather than to medical, factors.

The most likely condition for a nursing home resident to be suffering from is dementia. The most severe medically ill patients, those who are moribund, are commonly those who are in the end stage of a dementing illness. In addition, many of the medical conditions seen, such as bedsores and contractures, are the result of immobility, enforced by the use of physical restraints and psychotropic drugs. As previously shown, over half of nursing home patients are demented, and their dementia is likely to be accompanied by behavior disturbance. They are also likely, as we have seen, to suffer from other psychiatric conditions.

The elderly are institutionalized, whether in the acute care general hospital or the nursing home, because of three sets of factors: socioeconomic, behavioral, and medical. The complexity of these interactions has not escaped the attention of researchers or government agencies.

MEASURING NEED FOR CARE

One answer is to ignore specific diagnoses and to measure function by means of a scale of activities of daily living (ADLs). Activities of daily living comprise just about everything we must do to keep ourselves alive and functioning independently—such as dressing ourselves and feeding ourselves and getting to work on time. ADL scales (Crook, Ferris, and Bartus, 1983) must consider many complexities. What somebody can do for himself or herself with prompting and supervision may not be the same as he or she actually does if left alone. Some individuals are waited on hand and foot to such an extent that they do not know how to boil an egg. ADL capacity may be limited by assigned sex roles, as in the case of a husband who does not know how to sew a button on a shirt. In some communities everyone needs to know how to drive a car, and in others everyone needs to know how to take the subway. Because of this, a separate category is often made of "IADLs" (instrumental activities of daily living). These are the more complicated activities, such as shopping or driving a car, that demand certain amounts of initiative and intellect. Other subcategories are sometimes made, such as "PADLs" (performance activities of daily living) referring to the more basic and physical tasks.

In addition to medical and psychiatric disabilities, there are financial, social, and other disabilities. Therefore, the geriatric literature contains several scales for even more comprehensive assessment. Versions of such scales are incorporated in the instruments used in assessing possible candidates for nursing home admission by preadmission screening (PAS and PASARR).

THE INFORMAL NETWORK OF CARE

The sick are helped to stay in their own homes by various professionals, such as visiting nurses and home aides. To an even greater extent they are helped by their families, particularly by the women in their families (Lyons and Zarit, 1999). The informal network of care also includes friends who drop in, and neighbors who watch out, stores that deliver, helpful cabdrivers, and concerned policemen. If one does a survey of patients in the community, it is surprising to discover the severity of sickness in those who are kept out of nursing homes. This often occurs at the expense of great strain upon members of an informal network of care, who breathe a sigh of relief and disappear into the woodwork when the patient in institutionalized (see Chapter 21).

THE ROAD TO THE NURSING HOME

Entering a nursing home is often described as being a more rational and organized decision-making process than it really is in practice. Some authors (Retsinas, 1989) pay due regard to the financial and emotional aspects of this process. People enter nursing homes from acute care general hospitals, from their own homes, or sometimes from other institutions.

Admissions from the Community

Those who enter the nursing home directly from their own homes tend to have fewer medical problems below the neck than those who come from hospitals, but tend to be more severely mentally ill. A young, able-bodied male who frequently calls the police because of imaginary intruders is liable to be institutionalized in a psychiatric hospital, but an elderly female who does the same is put in a nursing home, often with a diagnosis of dementia. Such a diagnosis can be backed up by one of the highly sensitive but nonspecific tests such as the Minimental Status Examination (Folstein, Folstein, and McHugh, 1975) and by the presence of cerebral atrophy on a CAT scan.

The family of a patient living at home will often telephone or visit a local nursing home to obtain information on admittance. This is not the official route, but is so common that nursing homes are well advised to delegate someone to answer such calls and begin the liaison with the family. In most cases this duty falls upon the social worker, but other staff members could also become familiar with the process. Families call the nursing home because someone is there to answer the telephone twenty-four hours a day, seven days a week. The social worker is not always available, so whoever is manning the switchboard could have the telephone number of the local office on aging and the Alzheimer disease society, which are good places to begin. Telephone numbers that the family will need to get their mother on Medicaid and to get a nurse to come to the house to fill out the forms could also be given to the family.

First, the family must enroll their mother in Medicaid. This is a hassle because it means going to the county or city social service department (i.e., the "welfare office") and waiting in line with the other welfare applicants. If she is too wealthy to qualify for Medicaid, they must reduce her funds before applying for Medicaid. It is best to seek a lawyer's advice for this process. Many lawyers specialize in "poverty law," which is the art of stripping assets so that the government does not know about them. It is sometimes helpful to preserve some funds in the mother's name. Keeping assets in her name may be useful in shopping for nursing homes, implying that the mother will be paying privately.

After consulting the lawyer and enrolling their mother in Medicaid, they will need a nurse to fill out a form stating that the prospective resident is sick enough to be in a nursing home. This "preadmission screening" (PAS) is normally a state requirement, even if the mother is entering the home as a private pay patient, because the states know that after the spend down they end up paying for everyone anyway.

Armed with these documents, the knowledgeable family can begin looking at nursing homes and talking to the person in charge of admissions (in most nursing homes this is again the ubiquitous social worker) and placing their mother on the waiting list.

Transfer from Hospital

A well-traveled road to the nursing home is through the acute care general hospital. (Transfers from mental hospitals have become rare.) The hospital is the antechamber to permanent nursing home placement. The hospitalization was the result of an acute physical illness in a previously healthy person that left her so severely and permanently disabled that only a lifetime of nursing home care could answer her needs.

For example, if a previously independent person suffers a stroke, acute hospital care is necessary at the early stages, and nursing home care is needed thereafter. Other scenarios are possible. One possibility is that when a person needs nursing home care, the easiest way to get in is to be hospitalized first. Stubborn elderly people are sometimes dealt with in this way. The patient's family will often begin by contacting a doctor. The doctor usually finds that not much can be done medically. Some doctors may be knowledgeable enough to tell the family at the first visit what to do next, but in most cases a series of telephone calls occurs, demanding that the doctor do something more, until one day the doctor tells them to bring the patient to the emergency room. There a diagnosis is made based, to some extent, on the symptoms. If the patient has been falling down, he or she will be checked for cardiac arrhythmias, be put on a Holter monitor, and will likely get a pacemaker. If the patient has been refusing to eat or drink he or she will be diagnosed as dehydrated and put on intravenous fluids. There is seldom any shortage of diagnoses in the elderly if one does enough tests.

The hospital is up against the DRGs (diagnosis-related groups), a provision of Medicare that limits payment according to diagnosis. The hospital may only get $500 for a dehydration (pacemakers are much better) so they will have a procedure to get the patient out and into a nursing home as quickly as possible. Hospitalization causes the elderly to lose their capacity to resist and their capacity to cope (Leipzig, 1998). The individual who walked into the hospital as a tough psychiatric patient leaves it on a gurney as an easy nursing home patient.

Preadmission Screening

Preadmission screening (PAS) for nursing homes is emerging as an important area of expertise in nursing practice. It is normally done by discharge planning departments when the patient is in a hospital.

When the patient is in the community, PAS is usually done by public health nurses (Lathrop, Corcoran, and Ryden, 1989) but registered nurses in private practice are also doing this work, and the complications created by the new OBRA regulations and PASARR have increased the demand for their services. PAS screeners normally need to be licensed in some way by the state agency responsible for Medicaid and nursing homes. Admission requirements dictated by Medicare and Medicaid are also usually applicable in practice to those who pay privately. This is partly because the owners may anticipate a spend down, but mainly because of legal requirements in most states (Miles and Tisdall, 1999). States run their own special training courses geared to OBRA requirements.

The state mandated training is usually training in how to fill out a state form, and this is as far as it goes. Obviously the person going out to do PAS is meeting with the prospective nursing home resident and the resident's family at a very strategic time. The nurse doing this work should, ideally, have a deeper knowledge and understanding of the situation than merely the ability to fill out a form. In private practice, the nurse who is being paid directly for this service will be giving better service if he or she is versed in the various alternative community resources available and can do a certain amount of social service work, guiding the family through the intricacies of the bureaucratic maze. Such a nurse should be familiar with the local nursing homes and service providers, and able to provide psychiatric and medical advice and counseling.

The Impact of PASARR

Essentially, the federal law now mandates that patients suffering from a mental illness other than dementia cannot be admitted to nursing homes except under certain narrowly defined conditions. In New York State, for example, the patient's physical needs are first assessed by the document called PRI, which determines the medical needs. Then the social, financial, and psychiatric factors affecting placement are determined by the document called SCREEN. This has been modified to comply with OBRA and PASARR.

It begins with a dementia qualifier. To qualify as demented (and thus eligible to go to a nursing home) the diagnosis must be based on "the documented findings of a neurological examination." (This is often interpreted to mean a CAT scan and a neurological consultation, although that is not really what the law says.)

Leaving aside the question of mental retardation, the next questions are meant to determine the presence of mental illness, as defined by OBRA. They are: Does the person have a major mental disorder? Has the person been in a psychiatric hospital within the preceding two years? Has the person been taking an antipsychotic medication for thirty days? Does the person present evidence of having a major mental disorder? If the answer is yes to any of these four, then the person is referred for a "level II screen," unless there is serious or terminal medical illness or need for postoperative care.

"Level II screen" involves a "mental illness assessment" by a psychiatrist. If the psychiatrist determines the patient is mentally ill (and not demented), then a doctor at the local state hospital decides if active treatment is needed. According to the federal law, this decision is supposed to be "based on" the psychiatrist's mental illness assessment, but it will probably be based on whether the local state hospital wants to take the patient.

Many exemptions in PASARR allow the placement of the mentally ill in nursing homes to continue. For example, presence of a medical illness may get a mentally ill patient into a nursing home. This "medical override" can come into effect if the patient is terminally ill, comatose, convalescent from a recoverable condition following hospitalization, or has severe lung or heart disease or certain progressive neurological diseases. Another exemption is for dementia due to Alzheimer's disease and related conditions. These are not, by some lexical quirk, considered mental diseases. Even at this point there is no actual prohibition on the nursing home taking such a patient. It is merely mandated that the patient is to get active treatment and that Medicaid is not going to pay for it.

The Initial Interview

In spite of all these screenings and forms it will often be found that the initial interview at the nursing home is the first one in which any professional discusses the patient's mental condition with the family. This is especially so when the patient has been in an acute care general hospital for (at least ostensibly) a medical or surgical condition. The discussion with the doctors there may have focused on the physical ailment.

A great deal may have to be accomplished at this initial interview. It is tempting to try to save time by interviewing all the family members together, but quite often this does not work out well. The feelings about a spouse are different from those about an elderly parent, however well loved. Even siblings can vary within a family in the intensity of emotional attachment. Mundane matters such as the spatial arrangement of corridors and nursing stations can affect how the family is grouped for interview, and should be given careful attention. The counsel of perfection would be to interview each relative separately; but, at the very least, spouses and children should be seen separately. It is beneficial to tactfully ascertain if the spouse is also demented.

It is always a good idea, as soon as possible, to get an idea of the family's expectations about prognosis and life expectancy. This can begin with general discussion of how old some of the present nursing home residents are, and what the prospects are of their mother reaching the age of the oldest resident. If one of the 2,000 Americans over 105 years old is present, she can be shown off, along with a discussion of longevity and life expectancy.

The distinction between nursing homes and hospitals should be made clear as early as possible. The primary role of the nurse in the health care team must be explained, and the channels of communication clarified. This can be done in an informational handout at the initial interview.

The time of admission to the nursing home is the best one for identifying the involved family (and the uninvolved family), the caregivers, the friends, the lovers, the ex-lovers, and the support network. This is not always simple or easy. We should know about the long-lost sister in Illinois, the estranged daughter in Kentucky, and the next-door neighbor who was the only one who really cared (see "the daughter from Ontario" in Chapter 7, p. 48). Their telephone numbers should be on the face sheet at the beginning, then kept up to date. The complexities of a family can be intricate, and the final days may see the denouement of ancient family dramas. This denouement should not be a surprise ending for the caregivers.

Is the Road a One-Way Street?

The patient who reaches the end of the road that leads into the nursing home will probably never return. Discharge from the nursing home may not always be welcome, especially if families have anticipated that the patient's future is now settled. Depression is an illness which may have a Lazarus effect. Sometimes an inactive patient with multiple mysterious physical ailments is placed into a nursing home after an inordinately long hospital stay. The patient's affairs are settled and the house is sold. The family, after much (or maybe not much) heart-searching, reconcile themselves to putting the family member in a nursing home and everything is squared away. If the illness is then recognized as depression and appropriately treated, the justification for nursing home care may evaporate. The announcement that the nursing home is no longer needed is not always welcomed on all sides.

PART III:
THE PROBLEMS

Chapter 10

Psychotropic Drugs

It may appear perverse to list psychotropic drugs under the heading of problems, but prior to OBRA '87 complaints such as "My mother looked like a zombie" were frequently leveled at nursing homes, and have not completely disappeared. Nursing homes are still accused of drugging their patients with heavy doses of tranquilizers and of overusing physical and chemical restraints. Much time and effort must go into countering the accusations and preventing the circumstances that might justify them.

The controversies and government restrictions center upon drugs producing a sedative effect. Antidepressants, usually nontricyclic (see Chapter 13), are now the most common psychotropic drugs used in nursing homes (Lasser and Sunderland,1998) but have generally escaped stigmatization.

SURVEYS

As far back as 1976, a survey of over sixty nursing homes by Glasscote and colleagues found that over half the residents were receiving psychotropic drugs on a regular basis, that fewer than 10 percent of these had a recorded diagnosis justifying use, and that "virtually none" had been seen by a psychiatrist. By 1980, nine major surveys were conducted regarding prescription drug use in the elderly. Almost all surveys stated or implied that the drugs are used more than they should be.

Burns and Kamerow (1988) studied practices in a sample of all nursing homes in four standard metropolitan areas. Of patients receiving psychotropic drugs, one-third did not have any justification in terms of the chart diagnoses or the information obtained by the interviewers. Half of this third were on antipsychotic medications. Sedatives and hypnotics were the most frequently misused drugs, and the use of a sleeping pill every night was the most common error. If there was a true indication for an antipsychotic drug, such as an established diagnosis of schizophrenia, then the dosage was often subtherapeutic. All the improper antidepressant dosages were subtherapeutic.

Beers and colleagues (1988) examined medication use in nursing homes in Massachusetts. They found that suboptimal choice of medication was common. Two-thirds of the nursing home patients had orders for psychotropic or hypnotic medications. One-third had orders written for antipsychotic drugs and one-fourth received them, yet very few were diagnosed as psychotic. Essentially, they concluded the drugs were being used as a chemical restraint.

Waxman, Klein, and Carner (1985) attempted an analysis of the institutional dynamics leading to excessive drug use. They suggested that the pressure stemmed from administrators who in turn felt pressured by the aides. The administrators believed that the aides would have an easier time if the patients were sedated. Ray, Federspiel, and Schaffner (1980) found that the typical heavy prescriber of tranquilizers was a rural general practitioner with a large proportion of his practice in nursing homes, in which he was the primary physician for most of the patients. He graduated between 1950 and 1959 and was not board certified. The authors suggested that the significance of the years of graduation may be that these were doctors who witnessed the advent of the antipsychotics in the days when they were being hailed as the new miracle drugs, and thus had a more benign view of them. Buck (1988) could not find any particular patterns of demographics determining medication prescribing, and did not find any tendency for larger nursing homes to be more likely to use psychotropic drugs.

Studies from outside the United States showed similar tendencies. Morgan, Gilleard, and Reive (1982) in Scotland, studied the use of hypnotic drugs in residents of homes for the elderly run by a county agency. Such homes correspond closely to board and care homes in the United States in regard to staffing, although they tend to contain sicker patients who might be in nursing homes in the United States. They found evidence that the phenothiazines were being given at night as hypnotics rather than to treat a primary psychiatric disorder. The most common hypnotics were benzodiazepines.

BACKLASH

Most of these surveys, as Burns and Kamerow (1988) pointed out, did not study sins of omission. They did not look for cases where psychotropic drugs were not used but should have been. This failure may be both a result and a cause of an assumption that the main problem in nursing homes is one of excessive use.

Peck (1989), based on "34 years of service in a large nursing home," found drugs indispensable for treating the demented who are "screaming, biting, kicking, and punching those around them" and claimed that with their correct use patients can be made "alert, responsive, and capable of social interaction."

Loving and caring children who keep their demented parents in their own homes will sometimes use these drugs, so the use cannot be entirely the result of malevolence and laziness by nursing home staff. Community figures suggest that pressure for sleeping pills and antianxiety drugs comes from patients themselves. Prien (1980) compared use inside the nursing homes with use in the community. He found that in the nursing homes 20 percent received neuroleptics (3 percent in the community), 7 percent antidepressants (2 percent in the community), 15 percent antianxiety drugs (17 percent in the community) and 35 percent sedative/ hypnotics (9 percent in the community).

THE IMPACT OF OBRA '87

It is likely that many of the studies described influenced the framers of OBRA '87. OBRA took a definite stand against antipsychotic drugs, perhaps beyond what the evidence justified. It specified, "Residents who have not used antipsychotic drugs are not given these drugs unless antipsychotic drug therapy is necessary to treat a specific condition" and that "residents who use antipsychotic drugs receive gradual dose reductions, drug holidays or behavioral programming unless clinically contraindicated in an effort to discontinue these drugs" (*Federal Register,* 1989, p. 14). HCFA guidelines for the surveyors implementing OBRA prohibit the use of psychotropic drugs "for the purpose of discipline and convenience and not required to treat the resident's medical symptoms" (HCFA, 1991, p. 48849).

Psychotropic drugs are now being used less, although about a quarter of a million nursing home patients still take them (Llorente et al., 1998). This may represent improved standards of practice or that the homes are finding it inconvenient to use psychotropic medications because of the many required forms. Psychiatric consultations are now likely when a psychotropic drug is used.

Some questions about the use of psychotropic drugs remain unanswered but the changes in their use are probably beneficial. In an open controlled prospective trial, Puroshottam and colleagues (1994) compared nursing home residents whose antipsychotic medicine was stopped with those who continued to receive the medicine. The withdrawals took place in the context of a program designed to reduce use of these medications in conformity with OBRA '87. Residents with a recent history of violent behavior or under treatment for psychosis were excluded. Several rating scales were used by multiple observers. The frequency of behavior problems did not increase, and many residents improved. The symptoms that improved particularly were blunted affect, tearfulness, motor retardation, and emotional withdrawal.

Terminology

To consider whether these charges against this class of drugs are justified, we must begin by examining the terms used. Tranquillizer is not really a medical term. Any drugs used to affect mind or mood is called a psychotropic drug. Drugs used in the treatment of severe mental disorder are called antipsychotics. Among those most commonly used in nursing homes are thioridazine (Mellaril), chlorpromazine (Thorazine), haloperidol (Haldol), and thiothixene (Navane). These drugs are also called "major tranquilizers" and "dopamine-blocking drugs." The first two are phenothiazines. A newer group of drugs are called "atypical antipsychotics."

ANTIPSYCHOTICS

The antipsychotic drugs were introduced in the 1950s to treat schizophrenia. At that time they were hailed as miracle drugs and, indeed, they merited that acclaim. Hitherto there had been no effective treatment for schizophrenia. The dosage in which they are used for treating young people with schizophrenia is many times greater than that used in nursing homes. Not every case of schizophrenia is cured, and we can still find cases of those who do not function and who wander around muttering and talking to voices (although some of these may not be taking their medication).

In schizophrenia, antipsychotics suppress delusions and hallucination. They produce drowsiness, which usually begins about two hours after they are taken and lasts for about twelve hours. Prisoners who have been forcibly given large amounts have complained of the lethargic drugged sensation. It is often difficult to persuade alert patients to take them on a long-term basis, but those who have been subject to alarming delusions and hallucinations and who have found these symptoms relieved by these drugs will be willing to take them. Sedative effects can be avoided by careful dose timing and titration.

Avoidance of sedation can be a mixed blessing. The absence of a chemical straitjacket effect is not always perceived as a benefit by the nursing home staff. The prescriber needs to be aware that some nursing home staff may actually want the patient sedated and may find it easier to deal with the complications of sedation and an immobile patient than with an active ambulant patient. Other staff (and more especially families) may perceive the patient as overmedicated.

Antipsychotic drugs in general do not impair memory and cognitive function as do the benzodiazepines and anxiolytic drugs that work on the same part of the nerve cell (the γ-Aminobutyric acid or GABA receptors). Indeed, in young patients with schizophrenia, memory may be apparently improved. This is because severely psychotic patients may not be willing to cooperate with memory tests (Jeste et al., 1999).

Adverse Effects

These drugs are very safe, in the sense that it is difficult to die from an acute overdose of one of them. The only acutely life-threatening adverse effect is neuroleptic malignant syndrome, characterized by high fever. This condition can be difficult to diagnose in the nursing home, where fever, agitation, and decreased levels of consciousness are common (Colón-Emeric and White, 1999).

Evidence that psychotropic drugs increase liability to pneumonia and choking is disputed. The drugs have been associated with falls and hip fractures in nursing homes. Since they reduce mobility, they may predispose to the medical complications of immobility. They can cause low blood pressure, especially standing up (postural hypotension).

Many of these drugs, at high dosages, produce extra-pyramidal symptoms (or "EPS") to varying degrees. Some patients develop acute dystonia, with arching of the back and clenching of the jaw. Milder cases can show parkinsonism, with slow shaking, a frozen zombie face, drooling of saliva, and a shuffling gait. These symptoms can often be helped by giving benztropine (Cogentin) or trihexyphenidyl (Artane) along with the antipsychotic. However, Cogentin in turn produces anticholinergic side effects, such as precipitation of glaucoma, retention of urine, and constipation, which can be especially troublesome in the elderly. When taken over a very long time antipsychotic drugs can cause lip and tongue movements, called tardive dyskinesia, which may be permanent. The elderly are especially liable to this.

"Atypical" Antipsychotics

The action of antipsychotic drugs is apparently related to their blocking of the action of dopamine in the brain, although their action on serotonin and other receptors may also be important.

Dopamine receptors are of several kinds, designated D_1, D_2, D_3, D_4, and D_5. It is the blockage of D_2 that mainly causes the neuromuscular reactions, and manufacturers have tried to reduce this blockage, producing a generation of antipsychotic drugs that are still referred to as "novel," "atypical," or "new" (although clozapine has been available in the United States since 1989 and risperidone since 1994). These drugs are less likely to cause parkinsonism and tardive dyskinesia. An increasing proportion, now about one-third, of antipsychotics prescribed in nursing homes are of these "new" types (Lasser and Sunderland, 1998).

Low starting doses are recommended with the new antipsychotics in the elderly although the range is not yet fully and exactly established. Suggested starting doses (per day) have been 6.25 to 12.5 mg for clozapine, 0.25 to .5 mg for risperidone, 1 to 5 mg for olanzapine, and 12.5 to 25 mg for quetiapine (Jeste et al., 1999).

"Atypical" Antipsychotic Drugs

	Effects likely to be of particular concern in nursing home patients
Clozapine (Clozaril)	Need for blood counts Postural hypotension and falls Constipation
Risperidone (Risperdal)	Not as completely free of parkinsonism as the other atypicals (Arenson and Wender, 1999)
Olanzepine (Zyprexa)	Postural hypotension and falls. Expensive
Quetiapine (Seroquel)	Cataract formation; Expensive

Psychotropic Drugs in Dementia

None of these drugs has been shown to improve memory or cognitive disabilities in dementia (Helms, 1985) but they have been extensively used in nursing homes to treat such symptoms complicating the dementia syndrome such as irritability, hostility, agitation, anxiety, sleep disturbance, delusions and hallucinations (Barnes et al., 1982).

DRUGS FOR MANIA

Lithium is a specific treatment for mania. It does not cause the usual antipsychotic drug side effects, such as drowsiness or parkinsonism. Blood levels and other blood tests are needed to monitor the dosage. In a nursing home setting such tests are relatively easy to arrange. Nevertheless, this drug's use in this population is not simple. Bushey, Rathey, and Bowers (1983) found that only four out of twelve nursing home residents remained free of side effects after five years on lithium, and that it was especially liable to cause shaking and confusion.

Other antimanic drugs have recently been introduced. These are not as specific as lithium, and were originally used in treatment of epilepsy. They are often used as medications of desperation in psychiatric conditions that have failed to respond to anything else. Valproic acid is the most common of these (see Chapter 17).

ANTIANXIETY AND HYPNOTIC DRUGS

Drugs that reduce anxiety and assist sleep have many effects in common with one another and with alcohol. These effects include liability to cause falls and impairment of memory. The effects on memory often include a slight immediate deleterious effect, a long-term damaging effect on the brain from high dosages, and acute confusion if stopped abruptly after being used for extended periods. Seizures and mental disturbance can occur during withdrawal. These similarities, in effect, are probably because all these substances act on the GABA (γ-Aminobutyric acid) receptor, which inhibits nerve cell activity.

The terms "minor tranquilizer" or antianxiety drug, refer to a group of drugs of which the first were phenobarbital and meprobamate (Miltown, Equanil). These two old standbys have now largely been replaced by newer ones belonging to the chemical class called benzodiazepines. These started off as chlordiazepoxide (Librium) and diazepam (Valium) but have proliferated, along with the profits of the drug companies making them. They now include clorazepate (Tranxene), flurazepam (Dalmane), oxazepam (Serax), temazepam (Restoril), alprazolam (Xanax), clonazepam (Klonopin), prazepam (Centrax), triazolam (Halcion), and lorazepam (Ativan).

There is little to choose among these drugs except in terms of length of action. Halcion and Ativan are particularly short-acting.

The Case Against Benzodiazepines

Unlike the antipsychotics, the benzodiazepines are quite pleasant to take and can be addictive. This is among the features that has led to restrictions on their use. Reluctance to assuage anxiety with a drug that gives an immediate subjective sense of relief may be a manifestation of the puritan ethic rather than entirely rational practice, but the elderly who take benzodiazepines do not function well (Ried, Johnson, and Gettman, 1998).

One result of the demonization of benzodiazepines has been the promulgation of rules and regulations about their use in nursing homes by HCFA. Whether these are justified or not the prescriber must be familiar with them. They are only allowed for short-term use, unless justification is heavily documented, and the government prefers short-acting ones to long-acting ones.

Nonbenzodiazepine Hypnotics

Many medications are used to evade OBRA restrictions while satisfying a perceived need for sedation or for sleep medication.

Diphenhydramine (Benadryl) is an antihistamine; it can be used in treatment of parkinsonism, and it causes drowsiness. Because it causes drowsiness it is sometimes used at night, as a hypnotic. Another multipurpose drug used frequently in nursing homes is hydroxyzine (Atarax), which can produce sedation and relieve itching.

Several antidepressant drugs have a sedative effect and are used in this way. The antidepressant trazodone (Desyrel) is commonly used, in effect, as a sleeping medication (Lasser and Sunderland, 1998).

As mentioned above, several of the older generation of hypnotics, such as chloral hydrate, barbiturates, and meprobamate, remain in widespread use and are encountered often in nursing homes.

RECOMMENDATIONS

When patients with lifelong histories of psychosis are in nursing homes, and the diagnosis of schizophrenia is well-established, most psychiatrists would agree that the patients should continue on their antipsychotic medications. Stopping them usually (although not always) results in a recurrence of symptoms of psychosis that are certainly disturbing to the caregivers, and probably distressing to the patient.

Most psychiatrists would also agree that these drugs have a legitimate use in paranoid states of the elderly, where elaborate and distressing delusions and hallucinations exist.

The biggest difficulties concern the use of psychotropic drugs in agitated states where no psychiatric diagnosis has been made. To a large extent, the use of drugs in these cases is determined by the need for compliance with OBRA.

One response to this has been that when the patient seems to need sedation, a mental health professional is called in. Some mental health consultations are being asked for as a formality to justify the use of the psychotropic drugs. It is then up to the mental health professionals to ensure that they do not automatically rubber-stamp medication prescriptions without making a genuine contribution to the patient's welfare. In these circumstances, the psychiatrist who holds back on prescribing sedative drugs faces much the same problem as the academically correct pediatrician who holds back on antibiotics. The desire for the drug may be so strong that arguments against using it are countered, and an adversarial stance can develop. The skills needed to prevent such developments are more psychological than pharmacological.

Diagnosis, Documentation, Dosage

Good clinical practice is the ultimate defense against all criticism, but compliance with regulatory agencies demands special attention to these three areas. Accurate charting of psychiatric symptoms is as necessary as that of physical signs, and psychiatric diagnoses must be as well justified as medical ones.

When no DSM-IV or ICD-10 diagnosis is on record, or the only such diagnosis is in the dementia or delirium category, then the target symptoms for which the medication is prescribed must be documented. Such target symptoms will warrant a revision of the MDS and triggering of a RUGS protocol. This will, in turn, necessitate documenting that behavioral interventions, as well as medication, have been tried, however strongly the staff feel that medication is needed.

The effectiveness of the medication on the target symptoms must be noted, and reasons given for any dosage that exceeds standard recommendations. A primary diagnosis of a nondementing DSM-IV or ICD-10 diagnosis such as schizophrenia or bipolar disorder will always justify appropriate medication, and the presence of any such conditions should be recorded if medication is continued indefinitely. In other cases government surveyors may expect to see written evidence that the effect of reducing or stopping the medication ("drug holidays") has been observed.

Chapter 11

Memory Loss and Confusion

Most people in nursing homes have lost, to some extent at least, the kind of mental abilities the human brain shares with computers, such as memory and ability to do arithmetic or play chess. The loss of these abilities correlates well with finding physical changes in the brain that can be seen under the microscope and accurately measured. In some ways, therefore, this is a very exact and scientific area of psychiatry. Nevertheless the terminology can be inexact.

THE TERMINOLOGY OF DEMENTIA

Confusion, in psychiatry, means being so mixed up as to be disoriented in space and time with inability to recognize family members (disorientation to person). Impairment of "cognitive function" usually means impairment of memory and of the intellectual capacity to do such things as simple calculations. "Organic mental syndrome" and "organic brain syndrome" are terms that were once used for dementia and delirium. They are out of style now, although the "organic mental syndrome" was still in the *Diagnostic and Statistical Manual of Mental Disorders* published by the American Psychiatric Association, up until DSM-III was changed to DSM-IV.

Delirium

Delirium is an old-fashioned word which has now returned to official favor, and is a recognized diagnosis in DSM. Many of the older of us never stopped using it, although for some years we were being told

93

that we were out of style and that the correct term was "acute brain syndrome" (or "acute exogenous reaction type," "acute confusional state," "toxic psychosis," or "metabolic encephalopathy"). In traditional medical usage, delirium was an acute state, but the current DSM-IV and ICD-10 definitions allow it to be used for prolonged states, thus blurring the distinction from dementia.

Those who are delirious have lost their awareness of the activity around them. The main point of distinction from dementia is that it is more acute in its onset, and does not last long. Vivid visual hallucinations, such as pink elephants or little green men, are no longer required for the diagnosis, but delusion, hallucinations, rapid fragmented speech, and restlessness are recognized as features. Between one-third and one-half of the hospitalized elderly are delirious (Lipowski, 1983).

The list of causes of delirium includes almost every medical illness in the book. It is a nonspecific symptom, like fever, which is not a diagnosis in itself, but demands a search for the medical condition causing it, as well as management of the symptom.

Alzheimer's Disease

Dementia is a more chronic situation than delirium; loss of memory is the hallmark. Other intellectual faculties (cognitive functions) are also lost. Dementia due to disease of the brain for which no cause is known is called a "primary degenerative dementia." Dementia associated with the microscopic brain changes descibed by Alois Alzheimer is called "dementia of the Alzheimer type" (DAT). Recently it has been frequently called "Alzheimer's disease," although Alzheimer described symptoms other than dementia associated with the brain changes. The only certain way to tell if Alzheimer's disease is present is by looking at the brain under the microscope after death. When a primary degenerative dementia occurs early in life it is called a "pre-senile dementia."

Vascular Dementia

Disease of the arteries supplying the brain may cause cutting off of the blood supply to a part of the brain. This part of the brain then dies, producing a softened area of dead brain tissue called an infarct.

The result may be to produce a stroke or dementia, or both. There is some doubt as to whether disease of the arteries inside the brain (cerebral arteriosclerosis) can cause damage without actually producing an infarct. Because of this there was a tendency to replace such terms as "arteriosclerotic dementia" and "hardening of the arteries" with the term "multi-infarct dementia." However, the pendulum of fashion has swung back and the present official term is "vascular dementia."

Infarcts can be seen by brain imaging techniques, such as computer assisted tomography (CAT) and magnetic resonance imaging (MRI). Another way of deciding between Alzheimer's disease and artery disease is to make a list of the patient's clinical signs of stroke and heart disease. Those who score high on such a list are assumed to be more likely to have multi-infarct dementia. Infarcts are found on the CAT scans of many dementia victims. Such cases are not usually referred to as having had a stroke if their symptoms were purely mental.

A stroke is usually defined in neurological terms. It causes a sudden loss of consciousness and paralysis of part of the body, usually one complete side (hemiplegia). It is possible, and indeed common, to suffer a brain infarct and have the brain changes of Alzheimer's disease. The sufferer from such a double set of brain diseases will probably be demented.

The amount of dementia due to Alzheimer's disease as opposed to cerebral artery disease has been variously estimated. No true population study has ever been done, but the general consensus is that Alzheimer's is more common. Ethnic variation is possible. Serby, Chou, and Franssen (1987) found that most of a group of demented American-Chinese nursing home residents they examined had multiple brain infarcts.

Alcohol-Related Memory Loss

Probably the most common dementia to improve in the nursing home is that resulting from alcohol or drug use. The alcoholic amnesic syndrome is sometimes said to be irreversible, but tends toward recovery with time and sobriety.

The alcoholic wet-brain may not be diagnosed, and may be admitted to the nursing home as a case of primary degenerative dementia.

Without access to alcohol, a gradual recovery takes place. Occasionally this recovery may be embarrassing in its completeness, since many of these are socially isolated males who present problems of management and placement that a nursing home is ill-equipped to handle.

An alcoholic, socially isolated man was hospitalized because of multiple medical problems resulting from his drinking. After treatment of his acute medical problems he remained disoriented in space and time, and needed assistance with his self care. Because of this mental state, he was transferred to a nursing home. Over the next few months in the nursing home he made further physical recovery and became fully ambulant. His memory and intellect progressively improved. He became obstreperous, demanding, and aggressive. Attempts were made to place him in a lesser care facility, but he was uncooperative, and it was difficult to find a place he would accept and that would accept him. Eventually he absconded, returning to the local skid row.

Rare Kinds of Dementia

Rare kinds of dementia are relatively ordinary in nursing homes. This is because the prevalence exceeds the incidence. Acute brain conditions, such as anoxia, poisons, and various kinds of encephalitis, leave victims who survive for years in a brain damaged condition. Herpes simplex encephalitis is probably the most prevalent of these.

Several "neurodegenerative" disorders, such as Gerstmann-Sträussler syndrome, Friedreich's ataxia, and multiple system atrophy attack young people, leaving them crippled and eventually immobile. Creutzfeldt-Jakob ("mad cow") disease is rapidly progressive, with myoclonus, involuntary movements, and mutism.

British and Swedish workers identify an entity of "frontotemporal dementia," which includes Pick's disease. Early behavioral symptoms, according to this group, include neglect of personal hygiene and grooming, lack of social tact, shoplifting, unrestrained sexuality, violent behavior, inappropriate jocularity, restless pacing, mental rigidity and inflexibility, overeating, food fads, excessive smoking and alcohol consumption, oral exploration of objects, clapping, singing, dancing, ritualistic preoccupations, hoarding, impulsivity, and "impersistence" (Lund and Manchester Groups, 1994).

The term "subcortical dementia" is sometimes used for the dementia associated with Parkinson's disease, Huntington's chorea, and the condition resembling Parkinson's disease called progressive supranuclear palsy. It is supposed to be less likely to show speech disturbance as an early symptom, and to be marked by a slowing of thought processes. Parkinson's disease overlaps with Lewy body disease, which is characterized by an onset of delusions and hallucinations, and sensitivity to the muscle-stiffness producing effects of neuroleptic drugs.

It is often of more practical diagnostic importance to clarify the kind and extent of disability than to arrive at the precise name of the entity. If, for example, communication is impaired, then the primary task of psychiatric assessment, a task that may involve all members of the treatment team, is often to clarify how much of this is mental and how much due to dysphasia or dysarthria.

HOW MANY OF THE ELDERLY ARE DEMENTED?

Since dementia is the major reason for nursing home admission, the statistics for prevalence are considerably influenced by whether nursing home residents are included, and community surveys may be misleading. In Hendrie's (1998) study of elderly African Americans in Indianapolis, the estimated rates of dementia were doubled if nursing home residents were included, rather than limiting the survey to those at home. Hoffman and colleagues (1991), in a European population survey, found 1 percent in the age group sixty to sixty-five were demented with the number doubling every five years, rising to 32 percent in the age group ninety to ninety-four, and more men than women in the younger age groups. American surveys usually show a higher incidence.

MEASURING MEMORY LOSS AND CONFUSION

Numerous scales have been devised to measure dementia, and no one can expect to be familiar with all of them. Essentially, all scales include asking about whether the subjects know where they are, what date it is, the name of the President, and so forth. The Folstein Mini-Mental State Exam is widely used but is not very feasible for patients with physical or eyesight limitations (Bettin et al., 1998) and lacks selectivity; that is to say it labels too many patients as demented.

Many of these scales are too elaborate and time-consuming, in spite of what their authors claim, to be routinely used in nursing homes; but it is probably a good idea for someone on the staff to be familiar with one of the scales and to record the result somewhere in the chart. An indication of which questions the patient could not answer such as "could not say his name" or "did not know her age" can be more informative than the bare numerical score.

Several writers have described schemes for staging progress or severity of Alzheimer's disease (Cohen, Kennedy, and Eisdorfer, 1984; Riesberg et al., 1982). The Global Assessment of Functioning Scale is described in DSM-IV for use with Axis V of the APA's official nomenclature.

Investigation of Memory Loss and Confusion

The search for treatable causes of dementia has normally been completed before the patient is admitted to a nursing home. In 1982, Sabin, Vitug, and Mark found that one-third of demented or disturbed patients had no mention of a neurological or psychiatric ailment in their nursing home records and that many of these had clinical problems that were potentially reversible. However, under OBRA regulations since 1987, investigations are to some extent mandatory before anyone with a dementia diagnosis can be admitted, and the home is thus a repository for investigated and untreatable cases of dementia.

Even after a preadmission dementia workup, the patients can develop an intercurrent illness, thus worsening an established mild dementia. Illnesses such as hypothyroidism should have been tested for before admission, but may also occur as fresh illnesses during a prolonged stay. (Current nomenclature would classify many such entities as delirium rather than dementia.)

The patient who has been plied with antianxiety and sleeping pills at home and who goes into acute delirium on hospitalization is a familiar figure. Sometimes this natural history is extended, especially if the hospital is free with its anxiolytic drugs, and it is not until several weeks in the nursing home that the syndrome is unmasked.

Memory loss caused by prescribed medication has recently been noted. The list of medications that can produce delirium is very long, but antibiotics are not included. Prednisone, digoxin, and many blood pressure medications have been cited as causing delirium. The difficulty is knowing how prevalent this is. A patient who is taking large amounts of medications, each of which has delirium as a rare side effect, may experience delirium when these medications are taken together.

The anticholinergic intoxication syndrome, and some of the large numbers of drugs that can give rise to it, have been reviewed by Molloy (1987). The special liability of the elderly nursing home patient to anticholinergic-induced delirium arises from several causes. These include the tendency to be on several different medications prescribed by different specialists. They are also liable to be taking older medications that have fallen out of favor and with which their present health care professionals may be unfamiliar. For example, they may (perhaps justifiably) take tricyclic antidepressants, such as amitriptyline (Elavil) and imipramine (Tofranil). However, Seifert, Jamieson, and Gardner (1983) were not able to show any dose-related relationship between confusion and the use of anticholinergic drugs in nursing home patients.

Flacken et al. (1998) measured serum anticholinergic activity by competitive blinding assay in terms of atropine equivalents and found that it correlated with both the presence and the severity of delirium, but they note that anticholinergic activity can arise from endogenous sources and is not necessarily entirely iatrogenic.

TREATMENT OF DEMENTIA

The magic memory pill is yet undiscovered. So far no medication has been proved to usefully improve memory and cognitive function in the primary dementias. The decision to initiate or to continue one of the medications with acetylcholine-like properties claimed to help Alzheimer's disease must be individual, and partly based on family wishes.

It is possible that what the French call "le brain jogging" may have a beneficial effect on memory in the elderly (Butler, 1998). The techniques of Reality Orientation (American Psychiatric Association, 1969) are based on this idea and are close to what common sense might suggest as methods to improve awareness. It is useful to have Reality Orientation or a related program in place, and to have someone specially trained and assigned to it on a permanent and ongoing basis. There is by now a respectable body of literature establishing it as a technique (Holden and Woods, 1988).

Beck (1998) has classified psychosocial and behavioral interventions for Alzheimer's disease into cognitive, functional, environmental, integration of self, pleasure-inducing, and family (see Table 11.1).

None of these methods cures dementia, and programs such as Reality Orientation cannot be shown to make measurable differences to anyone's memory, but they show that a frontal assault on dementia is being made. They boost the morale of staff and families, and probably of patients.

TABLE 11.1. Psychosocial and Behavioral Interventions for Alzheimer's Disease Patients and Their Families

Types of Intervention	Examples
Cognitive	Mnemonics; lists and calendars; reality orientation; techniques from early childhood teaching
Functional	Independence-promoting strategies to use residual skills for eating and dressing; prompted voiding; exercise regimes and walking; sleep regimes
Environmental	Variations in noise and light levels; way-finding cues
Integration of self	Reminiscence; group therapy
Pleasure inducing	Pet therapy; recreational therapy
Family	Support groups; respite care; counseling

Source: Beck, 1998.

Family support groups and associations such as the Alzheimer's Association are another example of a valuable service for the demented, which cannot be shown to measurably improve their cognitive function. Programs such as "friendly visitors," which seem to improve morale, fail when it comes to any measurable effect on memory (Denney, 1988). However, it must not be assumed that all treatment is futile, or that they do not need a high level of care.

Statements by those who do not wish to have the demented in their facilities are often prefaced by the phrase "all she needs is. . . ." This conveys the message that looking after the demented needs something less than full medical and nursing care, and something less than full psychiatric care, and that such care is "only custodial." In fact, when psychiatric institutions set aside areas for the demented they find they need additional medical and nursing services. Most dementia units in nursing homes have had higher staffing levels than regular nursing home units, although a dementia unit should be able to make the medical nursing interventions needed for its residents more efficient. Stevens and Baldwin (1988) review the literature on the impact of nursing care and show that the demented require substantial nursing time, even though the beneficial results of this increased time are difficult to measure.

Should the Demented Be Segregated?

Most surveys show the demented make better progress when housed in segregated units, in terms of maintaining ADLs and family satisfaction, and that they do better in purpose-built units (Grant and Sommers, 1998). Patients who were regarded as uninteresting impediments to real medical care when scattered among others, now become the special object of concerned attention. Behaviors characteristic of the demented can be tolerated and dealt with more effectively when they are expected.

A specialized dementia unit should have some architectural or structural features to deal with wandering (not necessarily locked doors) and with agitated or violent behavior. One simple requirement is space. Access to an area for free ambulation in the open air can be most helpful for wanderers. Plenty of space is also the single most effective method for dealing with violence. A big old-fashioned state hospital ward can be ideal, and it is hoped that not too many of these will be demolished in the name of progress without thought to their possible uses.

The environmental adaptations were the most pronounced distinctions of the special units surveyed by Wiener and Reingold (1989). Obviously purpose-built facilities with special architectural features will be expensive initially. In some cases they have also been expensive, subsequently, because the special architectural features have not been as durable or practical as was anticipated. One Alzheimer unit designed specifically by one of the world's leading architects resulted in many of its features being unsuitable for demented patients (Berger, 1985).

Prior to establishing a specialized dementia unit, staff must receive special training. The primary medical care should be provided by a doctor whose main interest is dementia, regardless of whether his or her nominal specialty is psychiatry, neurology, or geriatrics. A psyhiatrist should monitor use of psychotropic drugs (Mace and Gwyther, 1989). Useful additional supports include a program for the staff that encompasses staff education rounds conducted by geriatric medical school faculty, and an interested medical staff. Caution is needed to prevent patients in a specialized dementia unit from being excluded from other activities in the facility (Benson et al., 1987).

A problem can arise regarding whether to mix the mildly demented with the severely demented. Their needs are not always identical. The severely demented, who have become unable to walk and need help with feeding, and are subject to pneumonia, may have problems much more similar to those of the medically ill. On the other hand, the mildly demented may have needs similar to those of the mentally ill or mentally retarded.

We know that one of the leading complaints that patients have about nursing homes is the other patients. The mildly demented may be upset by the severely demented. Although it might seem that the specialized unit offers the chance of higher quality care, families may not want their relatives to be in it. They may be able to ignore or deny their relative's dementia as long as he or she is in a medical setting, but the dementia unit forces them to acknowledge the nature of the illness. They may also fear that the emphasis on behavioral problems will lead to the neglect of medical problems.

It has been difficult to prove any advantage for separate dementia units by controlled trials (Ohta and Ohta, 1988). This may be because it is difficult to find adequately matched controls within the same nursing home. The treatment of dementia is a losing battle, so that successful recoveries cannot be pointed to as evidence of the advantages. In many trials of treatment of dementia, the best that can be done is to demonstrate a slowing down of the progress of the illness.

It might be thought that a dementia unit would be difficult to staff because dementia is an extremely challenging illness. However, many who have been frustrated by caring for the demented on a general floor will become enthused by the feeling that now they can finally help these patients. This enthusiasm may be felt at all levels, in spite of the fact that dementia must be considered, in some respects, an untreatable illness. The prospect of taking part in research is often an inducement, especially for physicians and psychologists. Specialization has a tonic effect in stimulating interest. There is no disease, no matter how bad the prognosis, where the patient cannot be helped a little by the ministrations of those who are experts on this condition.

To some extent, the creation of specialized dementia units brings the wheel full circle. It recreates the mental hospital, but this may only be a belated recognition of fact.

Autonomy and Decision Making

The problem of the legal decision-making capacity of the elderly is often solved by assuming that they have none. Their consent to being in the nursing home is assumed, even if they vigorously and repeatedly say they do not want to be there. If, for example, a demented man arrives at a psychiatric inpatient unit, then, in most jurisdictions, a decision has to be made as to whether he should be committed involuntarily, if he is unable to sign for himself. If, however, the same patient is brought on a gurney to a nursing home, then there is no provision for consulting his wishes.

An interesting example of this assumption is discussed in a paper by Crane, Zonana, and Wizner (1977) about Connecticut Valley State Hospital. They describe reviewing a group of involuntarily detained patients in the light of the Donaldson decision. This was a legal decision stating that nondangerous mental patients could not be kept in a state hospital against their will without specific treatment. In about 25 percent of the cases, they recommended transfer to a nursing home because of the patient's high degree of disability. Apparently, they felt that, if the patients were unable to decide whether they wanted to be detained, then they could legitimately be shipped off to a nursing home regardless of previously expressed wishes, because now their wishes could not be consulted.

Questions of consent to treatment are usually dealt with in the same pragmatic manner as consent to being in the nursing home. Procedures such as catheterization and tube feeding are done without signed consent. When signed consents are needed, the usual procedure is to assume that the patients are competent if they are signing for what the doctors advise. There are further ramifications as far as major operations are concerned, but these will seldom involve the nursing home. (DNR orders and living wills are further discussed in Chapter 20.)

Matters of competence to handle money involve state laws. All states have provisions for signing over power of attorney. Such powers of attorney normally become invalid when the signatory becomes incompetent, unless they are specifically "durable" powers of attorney.

Use of tobacco and alcohol in the nursing home involves questions of patient autonomy, especially when the resident is under treatment for an alcohol or tobacco-related illness. Should the use of these substances be treated as a psychiatric illness? How justified is the home in acting to prevent their use? In demented nursing home patients the dangers from the use of cigarettes is as much from fire as from tobacco-related illnesses.

Leff and Harper (1998) describe a patient with bilateral above-knee amputations and hemiplegia: "He smoked cigarettes in bed, often refused to bathe, insisted on voiding into an urinal in the dining room, and made sexual advances to female staff members and other residents" (p. 439). He bought himself a motorized wheelchair that he used to go out and obtain alcohol and "while intoxicated his baseline personality was accentuated" (p. 439). The authors discussed the ethical questions that arose from the nursing home should prevent him from using his wheelchair.

One solution in such a situation might be to hospitalize the patient as a psychiatric case, on the grounds that he is dangerous to others. In practice, the usual difficulty about committing from a nursing home to a mental hospital is finding an institution that will accept the patient. When the state hospital refuses to accept a dangerous or violent patient, then an independent psychiatric consultation should, if available, be obtained, and it should be placed on record in writing that adequate application has been made. It should be realized that some symptoms that seem obviously psychiatric in nature and "belong" in a mental hospital, can just as well be managed in a nursing home. Some unpopular behaviors are just as obnoxious wherever the patient is located. One sometimes hears the plea that a certain patient should be in a mental hospital because the loud shouting "wakes up our other residents." However, this patient is just as liable to wake up the residents of a mental hospital as of a nursing home.

HEAD INJURY

Some of the issues about long-term care for head injury victims are further discussed in Chapter 19. Cognitive impairment is sometimes the major or only problem for such patients and the question then arises as to whether they can be diagnosed as suffering from dementia and thus be placed in nursing homes. If the injury occurs in childood, before the age of full development of speech and intellect, then a dignosis of developmental disorder can be made. Dementia is ordinarily thought of as being of gradual onset and progressive in nature. The ICD-10 description seems to specify this. An entity of "dementia due to head trauma" is recognized by DSM-IV. Although these dagnostic quibbles may seem academic, they can become of practical importance when disputes arise over placement.

MENTAL RETARDATION

In one sense, almost all the mentally retarded in the state institutions reside in nursing homes. The Miller amendments to the Social Security Act provided for two levels of care. The Intermediate Care Facility (ICF) was intended to provide a rather less intense level of care, although still with RN or LPN availability twenty-four hours a day. The term "Intermediate Care Facility" disappeared from official use under OBRA, except in the one case of the ICF-MR, which was maintained for institutions for the mentally retarded (Levenson, 1989).

The ICF-MR was to be a state-run facility, giving care at a nursing home level, and with the residents paid for by Medicaid, as long as it met the Medicaid standards for a nursing home. In fact, certain special criteria needed to be met by the ICF-MR, which were different from those for the ICF- general (Redjali and Radick, 1988).

Naturally, states leaped at the chance to get the federal money. State facilities for the mentally retarded were rapidly converted to ICFs. By 1986, there were 144,000 residents in ICF-MRs (Lakin et al., 1989). In the event that a mentally retarded person needed care at a hospital level, no provision any longer existed for him or her. Thus victims of severe neurological handicaps and those with severe behavioral problems became orphans of the storm.

Several policies were adopted to deal with these orphans. Some of them were accommodated in the ICF-MRs, in spite of the high intensity of care they needed. Many of the behaviorally disturbed were discharged and then refused readmission, on the grounds that they were psychiatric cases. The psychiatric hospitals would refuse to admit them on the grounds that they were mentally retarded. They ended up in various places, including the streets, the jails, the adult homes, and the nursing homes.

The mentally retarded are thus often housed under the same financial arrangements as nursing home patients. This may be in an ICF-MR run by the state in the same place as the former state school, or whatever it was called. In some states there are privately operated ICF-MRs.

Some states have obtained waivers to get Medicaid funding from the federal government to subsidize group homes. Group homes have the advantage of reducing stigma, and provide to some extent the feeling that the mentally retarded are not really medically ill, but group homes are about the most expensive way of providing care (Utah State Auditor, 1998). In some cases, they may be in a regular nursing home. This is often the fate of those with severe neurological handicaps. In this discussion the concern will be primarily with those in the regular nursing homes unless otherwise specified.

Strictly speaking, housing the mentally retarded in nursing homes may be illegal, because Alzheimer's disease and dementia are not given any specific mention in the sections on mental retardation in OBRA '87 and, therefore, the prohibition against admission to a nursing home applies to the mentally retarded even if "dementia" is also diagnosed.

Prevalence in the Nursing Home

The intelligence quotient (IQ) is one of the oldest of mental measurements, and is so well-established that psychologists have not been able to persuade the public to replace it with anything more sophisticated. The scoring is fixed so that scores have a "normal" distribution. This means that 1 percent of the population will have an IQ of less than 70, and this is often taken as the definition of mental retardation. Of these, 25 percent are in institutions of some kind, and between 1 and 1.5 million are aged over fifty-five (Howell, 1986).

The mentally retarded in the nursing homes are predominantly those with multiple handicaps and usually find their way there via the acute care general hospital. What often happens is that a well-intentioned judge takes a look at the state institution and orders it to get rid of its patients. They are then discharged into lesser care institutions such as group homes, which are often prohibited against caring for physical illness, or lack resources to do so. Thus, as soon as a resident develops even a cough or a cold he or she is hospitalized. The ICF-MRs may also hospitalize their sickest patients. The acute care general hospitals convert them into nonambulant patients, who are then judged to be in need of nursing home care.

Risks

What are the risks to the mentally retarded of being in the nursing homes? One is the loss of their previous outside day activities. If the nursing home is being paid for by Medicaid, then funding may be cut off for attendance at outside programs because Medicaid is supposed to be paying for twenty-four-hour-a-day care. Thus, a mentally retarded person may be banned from the program he or she previously attended.

Overmedication is another risk. Within the ICF-MRs, widespread use of psychotropic drugs has occurred in the past. This may not have been all misuse. The mentally retarded are as liable to such illnesses as schizophrenia or manic depressive illness as the rest of us. Some of these illnesses may be helped by the right medication. Many of the lifelong misplacements in institutions for the mentally retarded have been of mildly retarded persons, who could have functioned in the community, but had the added handicap of mental illness. The recent tendency has been for fewer psychotropic drugs to be prescribed for the institutionalized mentally retarded. Poindexter (1989) found one-third of the residents in one ICF-MR receiving these drugs in 1979 but only one-tenth of the same cohort receiving them in 1987. The exact indications for antipsychotic drugs in the mentally retarded are not well defined, and the drugs can often be discontinued without adverse effects (Ahmed et al., 2000).

Overmedication of the mentally retarded can occur with anticonvulsants as well as with antipsychotics. When treating alert and mentally normal epileptics it is common to find that there are certain anticonvulsant medications that they refuse to tolerate, even with carefully monitored blood levels. They often will complain of neuro-psychiatric symptoms, such as drowsiness, dizziness, or feelings of being "drugged." Such patients will sometimes forego complete sei-zure control, rather than put up with the side effects of the medica-tion. One-tenth of elderly nursing home patients take anticonvulsants (Lackner et al., 1998). The mentally retarded in nursing homes are not usually articulate or powerful enough to voice their objections. The risk/benefits ratio of eliminating seizures versus side effects must be different in the nonambulant nursing home resident. They do not drive cars or operate heavy machinery but, on the other hand, sta-tus epilepticus can be fatal and might, in theory, lead to further brain damage.

Alvarez (1989) found that, in many cases, the antiepileptic drugs could be withdrawn without any relapse of seizures. He withdrew mentally retarded patients who had not experienced seizures for three years or more, effecting a very slow withdrawal. Almost half had no further seizures. If seizures recurred, he resumed treatment with one drug rather than automatically reintroducing two drugs.

A subtle hazard for the adult mentally retarded is the medicali-zation of the regime, which is liable to take place in a nursing home. Many of them tend to be hypochondriacal and they will readily re-duce their capacities for activities of daily living and center their lives around medications. In a nursing home the medical type activities, such as handing out medications and taking blood pressures, are given priority. The normal regime often involves speeding up the work of the day by helping the slow and clumsy to dress and bathe rather than doing such things for themselves. Reports on tempera-tures and pulse rates are considered more vital than reports on mood and self-reliance. Those with cerebral palsy are especially at risk from being put to bed, where they develop contractures and can lose the ability to walk. Nevertheless, the atmosphere of a nursing home can sometimes be better than that of the older large state institutions for the mentally retarded.

A sixty-five-year-old mildly retarded woman, who had been able to read and write and travel by bus, was discharged to family care from a state institution. She suffered two spells of unconscious-ness and she was put on 300 mg per day of phenytoin (Dilantin). Her behavior became erratic, and she was put on haloperidol

(Haldol). She developed a fever and vomiting and was hospital-ized. Metoclopramide (Reglan) was added to the Haldol, and the resultant dystonia was treated with benztropine (Cogentin). The Cogentin caused urinary retention, and she was catheterized con-tinuously, with the ensuing infection being treated with antibiot-ics. She became nonambulant and unable to communicate. She was discharged from the hospital to a nursing home. In the nurs-ing home her medication was gradually stopped, and her ambula-tion and speech returned. However, it was not possible to restore her to her previous level of independence.

Selzer, Finaly, and Howell (1988) compared elderly mentally re tarded nursing home residents with those living in other settings, which they categorize as "community-based." They found that the nursing home patients were less mobile (which may have been either a result or a cause of their nursing home placement) but otherwise had fewer medical and behavioral problems, although they were more likely to be medicated for psychiatric problems. The nursing home residents were less likely to receive vocational services, com-munity skills training, support from family members, or to engage in social and recreational activities with friends.

Once a mentally retarded person is put into a nursing home, he or she will probably stay there for life. This is especially tragic for such patients as the fully ambulant with Down's syndrome, who are iso-lated among the elderly without access to enjoyable outside activities and group interaction with their peers. Special programs for the el-derly mentally retarded have been developed in a few centers but are still few and far between.

The mentally retarded should commute from the nursing home to another place for their daytime activities, preferably by public trans-port. This has a normalizing effect and improves their morale. If there is a problem with funding such outside activities, then a strong pa-tient advocate should be recruited. This can usefully be a family member who votes in the constituency of the local state legislator, or a chapter of the Association for the Help of Retarded Citizens <www.ahrc.org>.

Chapter 12

Delusions and Hallucinations

Officially dementia is the only psychiatric illness that qualifies for admission to a nursing home, and the diagnostic hallmark of dementia is loss of memory and cognitive functions rather than delusions and hallucinations, but, in fact, delusions and hallucinations are frequent in nursing homes. If we follow cases of dementia forward, we find that delusions are absent in the early stages (of course, this may be tautologous, because the presence of delusions with only slight cognitive impairment may lead to a nondementia diagnosis). Demented patients with delusions deteriorate more rapidly than do demented patients without delusions.

Fleeting delusions and hallucinations in delirium are common. In some cases of dementia, memory loss can lead directly to one kind of delusion. This kind of delusion is sometimes called secondary delusion (although the nomenclature is not standardized). I call it the "Scotch tape and scissors" type of delusion, based on my own domestic experience. In some families, when the father cannot find the Scotch tape or scissors, he yells at the kids for taking it, until he finds it in the place where he put it. This transitory delusional experience based on memory loss is magnified in the severe memory loss of dementia, and can result in severe behavior disturbance.

Secondary delusions may center on money, with scrutiny of bank books and delusions of being stolen from. In these money-focused cases, the distinction is not as clear between elaborate persistent paranoid delusions and simple transitory delusions secondary to memory loss.

DELUSIONS IN DEPRESSION AND MANIA

The delusions of severe depression and mania reflect the mood disturbance that is present. Severe depression is characterized by delusions of guilt, poverty, and impending disaster. The prevalence and clinical features of depression in the nursing home are further discussed in Chapter 13.

SCHIZOPHRENIA IN THE NURSING HOME

Schizophrenia in all its forms is usually first diagnosed in young adults and its victims tend to die young. The schizophrenic patient in the nursing home is not usually regarded by the staff as particularly difficult. Patients with schizophrenia may be delusional and mutter to themselves, but they may remain fully ambulant, continent, and able to dress and feed themselves. If fact, one concern may be that they do not need the intense level of care required to justify reimbursement at a nursing home. As we have seen (Chapter 3), some of those discharged from the mental hospitals ended up in nursing homes, although there is disagreement as to how frequently this occurred. Currently, a common route into the nursing home is from a board and care home via a general hospital, as evidenced in the following case.

A seventy-one-year-old patient was seen in psychiatric consultation in a nursing home because of being "very moody," and accusing people of poisoning her. She sometimes interrupted eating to suddenly physically attack another resident. She had come to the nursing home from a general hospital following treatment for pneumonia and before had been in an adult home. Telephone calls and searches of old records revealed that before being in the adult home she had spent several years in a state mental hospital and had been on haloperidol (Haldol). In the nursing home, parkinsonism had been noticed and she had been given carbidopa-levodopa (Sinemet). She was independent in all her activities of daily living, except that she sometimes deliberately wet her bed.

On interview she appeared alert, ambulant, emaciated, and vigilant. She described herself as feeling "very good" but was hostile and suspicious. She refused to answer questions directly about her memory and orientation, giving such replies as, "I'm a princess" and "I don't tell my age." She said, "I am married. I have a husband and children downstairs." Sometimes her speech became complete gibberish and was interrupted by shouting, muttering, or laughing.

Compared with those retained in mental hospitals, sufferers from schizophrenia in nursing homes are less likely to show anger and aggression and positive symptoms. They are more regressed in their activities of daily living (Harvey et al., 1998). A similar regression is often seen when a schizophrenic patient is moved from a board and care home to a nursing home; Le Corbusier's dictum is often reversed, and we make the discovery that more is less. The focus on the nonpsychiatric medical condition is associated with a willingness to do things for the patients that they were previously able to do for themselves. A marked benefit to physical health in the nursing home is that smoking is stopped. Schizophrenics are heavy cigarette smokers and this may be the cause of early death (Kelly and McCreadle, 1999).

LATE PARAPHRENIA

In Bleuler's definition of schizophrenia "primary disturbances of perception, orientation, or memory are not demonstrable" (Zinkin, 1950, p. 9). Bleuler and Kraepelin could find no organic disease of the brain in such illnesses as mania, depression, and schizophrenia. This led to illnesses such as dementia and delirium being called "organic" with the implication that other psychiatric conditions were not due to physical disease of the brain. This question of a divide between "organic" and "functional" mental illness has caused some convoluted terminology to develop, because it is no longer politically correct to make the distinction, and yet some kind of divide exists. DSM terminology refuses to separate some mental diseases as "organic," although the *International Classication of Diseases* (ICD) still allows it. The difficulty is especially evident when we talk about the paranoid symptoms of old age. Older writers, and some recent ones

(Roth and Kay, 1998), ask whether the paranoid symptoms of old age are manifestations of an "organic clinical syndrome."

The question posed by these writers was whether paranoia in old age is the same as schizophrenia, and whether it indicates the presence in the brain of visible changes, such as the senile plaques and neurofibrillary changes that Alois Alzheimer saw under the microscope in the condition now named after him.

If an elderly person has positive symptoms of schizophrenia (delusions and hallucinations) and also suffers memory loss and cognitive impairment, then does this mean that the schizophrenia symptoms are due to a brain condition such as Alzheimer brain changes or vascular disease? Almeida (1998) would classify such a case as "Type B late onset schizophrenia" (see Table 12.1). On the other hand, Jeste, Palmer, and Harris (1998) maintain that, adhering strictly to DSM nomenclature, the diagnosis should be "psychosis secondary to a general medical condition" (p. 346).

The younger schizophrenic patient is more likely to be male with negative symptoms (such as withdrawal and apathy). The older schizophrenic patient is more likely to be female with persecutory delusions (Pearlson et al., 1989). Older patients are more likely to be demented and to have Alzheimer-type brain changes or cerebral arteriosclerosis.

TABLE 12.1. Almeida's Classification of Late-Onset Schizophrenia Clusters

	Type A	Type B
Cognition	Impairment constricted to cognitive extra-dimensional attention set shifting and planning	Generalized cognitive impairment
Positive symptoms	Frequent and severe, with particular complex psychotic symptoms, such as first-rank symptoms of Schneider	Symptoms tend to be simpler and less complex
Negative symptoms	Uncommon	Uncommon
Neurological signs	Higher score than normal subjects	Frequent and more severe
Neuroimaging results	Mild enlargement of lateral ventricles	Relative cerebral atrophy; more widespread signs of cerebrovascular disease

Source: Almeida, 1998.

Is this merely an academic issue? It can have practical effects on reimbursement and placement, and can affect prognosis.

The prognosis of completely nondemented elderly patients who develop delusions is disputed. In some studies they have shown no particular tendency to become demented. Holden (1987) studied all the cases of paranoid illness in the elderly in a well-studied area of London, following them for ten years. These cases were carefully diagnosed at the beginning, so as to make sure that there was no evidence of memory loss and no trace of dementia. However, after three years, over one-third had become demented. Different conclusions have been drawn from this study. Obviously, some overlap occurred due to chance. The number increases in any population with Alzheimer's disease as it is followed for longer periods.

PHANTOM BOARDERS

Phantom boarders are a subcategory of delusions which have a distinctive pattern (Mikkilineni, Garbien, and Rudberg, 1998). They predominantly occur in elderly women living alone. The victim says she is being persecuted by strangers who enter her house at night. They may enter the home and take up residence there, have parties, play loud music, and generally make a nuisance of themselves (Rowan, 1984). The victim may call the police or family or landlord to evict the intruders. She can see them in three dimensions; they whisper and talk to her. Tactile sexual hallucinations are remarkably common. Some degree of cognitive impairment is usually present, although this may be mild. Perhaps a slight weakness of reasoning power is necessary for the victim to be convinced of the reality of the intruders. The boarders seldom follow the patient outside her home; it is therefore unusual to find them in nursing home patients, although the presence of phantom boarders may have led to institutionalization. Sometimes the patients are hospitalized, placed on psychotropic drugs, lose their capacity for independent living, and are then permanently placed in a nursing home with a diagnosis of dementia.

RELEASE HALLUCINATIONS

Release hallucinations occur in the blind or the deaf, especially when the onset is sudden and the handicap severe. Mentally alert patients can usually recognize that they are not veridical, and they are not helped by antipsychotic medications. In young patients, their origin in sensory deprivation is usually obvious. In the presence of age-related cognitive impairment, diagnostic difficulty can arise. Many of the paranoid elderly are deaf, but they are seldom helped by hearing aids or otological intervention.

MANAGEMENT OF DELUSIONS AND HALLUCINATIONS

Antipsychotic medications are now the primary psychiatric method of dealing with psychotic symptoms. However, this resource has limitations in the nursing home. The use of antipsychotic medications is, rightly or wrongly, circumscribed by the governmental regulations described in Chapter 10. Other limitations are part of the general difficulties in using medications in the elderly and physically ill. By the very nature of paranoia, its victims will sometimes refuse medications.

Measures other than medication include change of environment and counterstimulation. Nursing home staff who are not accustomed to handling psychotic patients will often ask mental health professionals for guidance in dealing with delusions. Questions are asked about whether to "go along" or to try to argue the patient out of the delusions. In response to such questions, a socratic rather than a didactic attitude is best. Ask the questioners what they have already done and how they find it works. Effective strategies should usually be encouraged. The task of the mental health professional is often to reassure and instill confidence rather than offer precise prescription of particular methods.

As mentioned earlier, being in the nursing home may itself be a therapeutic change of environment in some cases of "phantom boarders." When the victim summons the neighbors and the janitor and the police in the middle of the night, these people often react by summoning the children. The children are told that they must "do something" about the situation, and this doing of something often eventually results in placing the family member in a nursing home. This measure can be quite effective in expelling phantom boarders. In fact, the remission of symptoms may cause a reimbursement problem because the severity of the condition no longer seems to justify a nursing home level of care.

Cooperative patients who hear voices can often deal with them by producing deliberate speech themselves, or by drowning the voices with conversation, or using Walkman-type earphones. Visual hallucinations sometimes can be dispelled by bright lighting.

Carstensen and Fremouw (1981) describe the management of a case of late-life paranoia in a nursing home resident without drugs. Staff were instructed to direct the conversation to another topic when she spoke of her fears, and to initiate conversations with her at times when she was not verbalizing her paranoid concerns. She was reassured that the staff understood that she believed her statements were true, and that they were there to help her. A therapist established a relationship with her by regular conversation. Misinterpretations of everyday events were corrected by, for example, opening a door to demonstrate that a supposed murderer was not lurking behind it. Conversations were focused on positive events, such as the patient's actions in helping other residents. The report is a most useful source for suggestions about dealing with such a case in a nursing home setting.

Chapter 13

Sadness and Depression

Some difficulties in discussing depression in nursing homes stem from the fact that "depression" describes a feeling that is familiar to most of us, yet we also use this word to describe an illness that can be treated by medication.

The thought of being placed in a nursing home is depressing for most of us. Many people say that they would rather kill themselves than live in a nursing home, and some do (Loebel et al., 1991). Despite this, the type of depression that one might intuitively expect from reaction to such circumstances ("adjustment disorder with depressed mood" in DSM-IV, §309.0) is not common. Perhaps this is because those who are most upset by the idea of going into a nursing home succeed in keeping themselves out.

Depression is often self-limited. The average length of an episode of depression was eight or nine months before modern psychiatric treatments (Lundquist, 1945), although widespread variation occurs, and some depressions last for years. Depression increases mortality in ways that are not fully understood, and nursing home patients suffering from depression are twice as likely to die (Kettl, 1999). Treatment can both shorten misery and save lives. Organic treatments have been especially successful.

DEPRESSION IN OLD AGE

Evidence that depression is more common in old age is conflicting. Some studies show that elderly females become less depressed as they grow older, but Murphy (1983) found that those who had previously suffered depressive episodes had them more frequently.

Depression in the elderly often presents with somatic symptoms. The elderly do not say they feel depressed. They say they feel ill, or bad, or "terrible," or "hurt all over." In many cases they complain of specific physical symptoms, such as pain in a part of the body. Depression at any age can cause weight loss, dry mouth, and constipation.

DEPRESSION IN THE NURSING HOME

Apart from just being a depressing place, a nursing home adds its own special hazards to depression in the elderly. The patient whose primary illness is depression is, in the nursing home, essentially in the position of being a psychiatric patient in a nonpsychiatric institution.

One special hazard of suffering from depression in a nursing home is that it may be ignored or misdiagnosed. Quiet, withdrawn, apathetic patients are often regarded as easy to deal with in the nursing home, and their quietness and apathy does not become a focus of medical attention.

Another hazard arises from the fact that depression in the elderly often presents with somatic symptoms. Geriatric depression has a way of mimicking physical illness, which also, of course, often coexists. In the medically oriented atmosphere of the typical nursing home, where the primary care physician is an internist or general practitioner, these somatic symptoms may be investigated and treated. If an elderly nursing home patient is investigated enough, several ailments will surface. The problem in the elderly is not usually so much making a diagnosis, as deciding which diagnosis to treat. When the victim is depressed, the wrong ailment is often treated.

Even if the illness is diagnosed, it may be mistreated. However, it is usually the identification, rather than the treatment of depression, that is a problem in the elderly. To some extent this presentation with physical symptoms is culturally determined by the fact that some of the elderly are not attuned to accept the reality of mental suffering. Even when they have been diagnosed with an acknowledged psychiatric illness, they may prefer to seek follow-up from a primary care physician rather than a psychiatrist (Habib et al., 1998).

DEPRESSION AND DEMENTIA

Depression in old age can be mistaken for dementia. Questions about memory and orientation may be answered only with moans and groans or silence. This can lead to the condition called "pseudo-dementia," which can occur even when the memory is intact. It is more subtle and difficult to detect that some degree of dementia may coexist with some degree of depression. The demented are less likely to report themselves as depressed than are those looking after them (Burke et al., 1998). In the nursing home it is common for depression to supervene dementia. Parmalee, Katz, and Lawton (1989) investigated whether depression could be accurately diagnosed among the cognitively impaired in a nursing home, and found that it could, although it may be difficult to recognize if the patient does not communicate well. It can be recognized by the presence of the so-called "vegetative" signs of depression, such as loss of weight and change in sleep patterns, but these are common symptoms in dementia anyway.

The diagnosis of a mood disorder superimposed upon dementia is most obvious in the mildly demented patient who is also bipolar (manic-depressive). In such a patient the staff will often learn to recognize the mood changes, and it can be well justified to treat empirically with antidepressants or mood stabilizers.

INCIDENCE OF DEPRESSION IN NURSING HOMES

A prevalence of about 3 percent of major depression in the community-dwelling elderly is often quoted, with figures for nursing home populations of a 15 to 25 percent prevalence and 13 percent annual incidence of new cases (Reynolds, 1994). Figures might be expected to vary depending upon whether a circumscribed definition of depression is used, or if the judgment comes from experienced psychologists and psychiatrists, or from a standardized questionnaire, but all three give similar results (Parmalee, Katz, and Lawton, 1989). Depression rates are higher than in the general population that they cite, but are similar to those found among geriatric medical outpatients.

Depression is especially prevalent among those recently admitted to nursing homes. This is a matter of practical importance. It is also interesting to speculate about why it should be so. It might be thought to be consistent with depression being due to transplantation and loss of familiar surroundings, but the increase is for major depression rather than adjustment disorder with depressed mood. Possibly some of those who are severely depressed on admission die or get re-hospitalized before they can become long-term nursing home residents, and this reduces the number of the severely depressed in the long-term population. Another possibility is that the illness leading to nursing home admission was a major depression that was mis-diagnosed and masqueraded as a chronic and untreatable physical illness or as dementia.

RATING SCALES

Numerous rating scales for depression have been devised. Despite voluminous literature, all have some disadvantages in the nursing home population. Their use in long-term care settings has been recently reviewed by Carrol (1998). Lengthy scales make exorbitant demands on staff time; scales that depend on verbal self-rating are unsuitable for demented or aphasic patients; scales that include items about physical symptoms are not specific enough for populations that include the physically ill. Obviously an item such as "Have you dropped any of your activities?" is problematic as a cue to depression in a stroke patient just admitted to a nursing home. DSM-IV specifies that depression can only be diagnosed on the basis of physical symptoms if the physical symptoms are not due to a general medical condition.

The MDS itself is probably adequate as a screening device, and in many homes the triggering of depression will lead to a psychiatric consultation or other assessment by a health care professional, who will give a specialized opinion. The Geriatric Depression Scale (Yesavage et al., 1983) is commonly used in long-term care facilities to evaluate residents who are cognitively intact, and the Cornell Scale for depression in dementia (Alexopoulos et al., 1988) is used for those with cognitive impairment.

TREATMENT OF DEPRESSION
IN THE NURSING HOME

The depressed elderly respond to both organic and psychological treatments of depression, although their response is slower and their likelihood of relapse greater than for the young (Reynolds et al., 1999). Electroconvulsive therapy (ECT) can be dramatically effective.

The aged, especially the very aged and poorly educated, often lack a vocabulary to describe their emotional states to the young and highly educated. This cultural barrier may be one reason that it is difficult to treat depression in the aged by any form of psychotherapy. Several other reasons, including discrimination, have been suggested as to why the aged do not receive much psychotherapy. However, very severe depression with limited ability to talk is always resistant to psychotherapy. Claims have been made on behalf of several varieties of psychotherapy, such as the cognitive therapy of Beck and the rational-emotive therapy of Ellis, to special efficacy in depression, but even these demand some sort of verbalization.

A nonorganic method of treating depression in residents of homes for the aging is described by Power and McCarron (1975). They used a control group and standardized rating scales and were able to demonstrate significant and lasting improvement. They describe their technique as "interactive-contact therapy," which largely seems to consist of friendly social interaction in fifteen half-hour sessions spread over several weeks.

Thompson and colleagues (1983) describe a method of overcoming the reluctance of the old for psychiatric treatment by describing their technique as "a course in coping with depression" and basing it on a "psychoeducational model" (p. 390). If effective, it is certainly economical of staff. Nonprofessional instructors were shown to be as effective as professional ones. Rating scales were used, but there was no untreated control group. The treatment consisted of six two-hour sessions with six to eight patients enrolled in each class.

ANTIDEPRESSANT MEDICATIONS

Most psychiatrists now favor organic treatments in severe depression in the elderly. Burns and Kamerow (1988) found that in nursing homes, antidepressants were the only category of psychotropic drugs for which the most common error was inadequate dosage. Partly as a result of such research, antidepressant medications are exempt from government inspectors' demands for medication reduction. Ten years after OBRA '87, a clear downward trend occurred in the use of most psychotropic drugs in nursing homes, but this downward trend was accompanied by an increase in the use of antidepressant medications (American Psychiatric Association, 1998) (see Table 13.1).

This increase in the use of antidepressant medications was due to several factors. They were not stigmatized as chemical restraints by OBRA. In fact, HCFA endorses the simple concept "antipsychotics bad, sleeping pills bad, antidepressants good," and takes pride in the fact that from 1987 to 1998 the use of antipsychotic and hypnotic drugs halved and the use of antidepressant drugs doubled (Haar, 1998). Prozac (fluoxetine) and its progeny were easier for non-psychiatric physicians to use than the tricyclics had been, and the drug companies that manufactured them and had them under patent launched (with good reason and in good faith) massive sales efforts.

TABLE 13.1. Trends in Nursing Home Use of Psychopharmacologic Drugs Before and After OBRA '87

| Time Period | Psychopharmacologic Drug Class | | | |
	Antipsychotic	Antidepressant	Antianxiety	Hypnotic
Pre-OBRA				
1974 (Government Study)	34.5%	7.0%	17.0%	37.5%
1976-1990 (Literature Studies	33.5%	12.5%	10.5%	17.0%
Post-OBRA				
1991-1993 (Literature Studies	15.5%	15.5%	11.5%	4.0%
1997 (Government Study)	16.0%	25.0%	14.0%	7.0%

Source: Kidder and Kalachnik, 1999, p. 58.

The side effects of the older generation and tricyclic antidepressants, such as amitriptyline (Elavil) and imipramine (Tofranil) are anticholinergic. They include dryness of the mouth, blurring of vision, constipation, and precipitation of such conditions as retention of urine and acute closed angle glaucoma, and acute confusional states. All of these are most likely to be problems for the elderly. Although it is now less common to initiate treatment with these drugs, many patients are still taking them. It is generally recommended (American Psychiatric Association Practice Guidelines, 1993) that antidepressant drugs should be continued for a long time, and nursing home residents who are taking and have benefitted from these established drugs should continue taking them.

THE "NEW" ANTIDEPRESSANTS

The adverse effects of the tricyclic antidepressants have led to the promotion, for geriatric use, of newer antidepressants with fewer anticholinergic properties, such as fluoxetine (Prozac), although some meta-analyses have found little difference between the "new" and the "old" in efficacy or adverse effects (Avorn, 1998). (The quotation marks for "new" are justified by the fact that Prozac has now passed its tenth anniversary on the American market.) They do not block acetylcholine as much as do the tricyclics and therefore cause less constipation, dryness of the mouth, and blurring of vision. They are less likely to affect the heart (Roose et al., 1998). They increase the amount of norepinephrine and serotonin at nerve cell endings (not necessarily the blood concentration). They do this by blocking the mechanism for mopping up excesses of these neurotransmitter substances, and are therefore called selective serotonin reuptake inhibitors (SSRIs).

About one-fifth of those who start antidepressant drugs stop them because of real or imagined adverse effects (Leipzig, Cummings, and Tinetti, 1999), but the "new" antidepressant drugs are so safe and easy to use that they are often initiated by primary care practitioners, leaving psychiatrists to deal with the nonresponders. Plasma concentrations of the drugs are higher in the elderly at any given dose. The clinical significance of this is not clear, but the dosages in the elderly are usually recommended to be lower (e.g., a starting dose of 10 mg daily for paroxetine). The most common side effects in the elderly have been drowsiness, weakness, loss of appetite, and sweating. Elderly patients are liable to develop low blood sodium.

Making a Choice

How does one choose among these "new" antidepressants? In practice, patient familiarity and choice is often a factor. Prozac is now a familiar and almost trusted name. This can work in its favor. On the other hand, many patients will have tried it and they or their families may insist it does not work. This gives an edge, deserved or undeserved, to the newer drugs.

Antidepressants vary in their liability to cause drowsiness. Mirtazapine (Remeron) and trazodone (Desyrel) are best known for this property, and are often used specifically for the depressed who complain of insomnia. Paradoxically, trazodone was the antidepressant least associated with falls in one retrospective study on nursing home residents, although the writers suggest that this is because it was used for less severe cases of depression (Thapa et al., 1998).

In a study of very old (average age 98) nursing home patients, Trappler and Cohen (1998) found no differences in response among fluoxetine (Prozac), sertraline (Zoloft), and paroxetine (Paxil), but noted that the medications were substantially less effective in those who were demented.

In trials not limited to nursing homes, Paxil has been found slightly more effective than Prozac in the elderly. Citalopram (Celexa) has been shown to improve cognitive function in patients with concomitant depression and dementia (Carrol, 1998). No difference could be shown between venlafaxine (Effexor) and Prozac (Costa e Silva, 1998). Two double-blind trials found Celexa, Prozac, and Zoloft about equally effective (Medical Letter, 1998).

Combining results in an arbitrary way, and without pretending a statistically sophisticated meta-analysis, the antidepressant drug league may be summarized in this way:

> *Least likely to be discontinued:* paroxetine (Paxil)
> *Most common reason for discontinuing in psychiatric trials:* not effective
> *Most common reason for discontinuing in general practice trial:* adverse effects

Least likely to cause withdrawal reactions: fluoxetine (Prozac)
Most common withdrawal symptom: dizziness
Most likely to need twice a day dosing: paroxetine (Paxil)
Most likely to need upward dose titration: sertraline (Zoloft)
Least associated with falls: trazodone (Desyrel)

In clinical practice, treatment of depression is always a mixture of psychology, drug use, social service work, family counseling, and common sense.

SUICIDE

The elderly take suicide more seriously than the young. They attempt it less often but once they have decided to do it, they plan more carefully, give less warning, and are more likely to succeed. Opportunities to intervene in a suicidal crisis are therefore fewer (Conwell et al., 2000). The incidence of successful suicide outside the nursing home is greatest among elderly males.

It is not unusual for nursing home residents to think of suicide (Uncopher et al., 1998). Abrams and colleagues (1989) found that six suicides occurred over a six-year period among patients over age seventy in New York City nursing homes. The mean age of those who killed themselves was eighty-five. Two were by hanging, two by jumping, and two by drug overdose. This was one-fifth of the rate among the rest of the population in the age group in New York City, so it has been argued (Borson, 1989) that this indicates that nursing homes provide some degree of protection against suicide.

Although depression is well-tolerated in the nursing home (even if not well treated), suicide attempts cause particular alarm, even if they are mild and non-lethal, thus the staff and administration will usually want the patient transferred to an inpatient psychiatric hospital setting.

Chapter 14

Anxiety and Sleeplessness

Dementia, major depression, and paranoid illness occupy more of the attention of geriatric psychiatry than do psychoneurotic and personality disorders. Inside the nursing home, especially, the tendency is for these disorders to be accepted as idiosyncrasies or diagnosed as physical ailments.

The word neurosis is now regarded as old-fashioned. What used to be called anxiety neurosis is now anxiety disorder, and it is divided into obsessive-compulsive disorder, generalized anxiety disorder, posttraumatic stress disorder, simple phobias, social phobias, agoraphobia, and panic disorder. We are perhaps accustomed to think of neuroses as a relatively mild form of mental illness, but in terms of loss of function and poor quality of life, the result can be as bad as in psychosis or organic brain damage and can result in nursing home placement.

Four areas that present particular difficulties in dealing with anxiety in the nursing home are hypochondriasis, the distinction between agitation and anxiety in dementia, the role of psychotherapy, and the use of antianxiety medications.

HYSTERIA AND HYPOCHONDRIASIS

Nursing home patients have many physical complaints for which no definite anatomical or chemical basis can be found. They also have a high death rate. This places a heavy burden on the practitioner for precise diagnosis, both medical and psychiatric, especially since it is now increasingly acknowledged that psychiatric conditions with physical symptoms are treatable. The tendency for depression in the elderly to present with physical symptoms has been discussed (Chapter 13).

Hysteria is another word that is supposed to have become obsolete. The person we used to call "hysterical" is now said to have a borderline personality disorder. The "hysterical neurosis" is now officially called dissociative disorder, or conversion disorder. The classical psychoanalytic theory about hysteria was that it was caused by a buried traumatic memory. According to this theory, the hysterical symptom was perpetuated by a secondary gain ("krankheitsgewinn"), that is to say, by some benefit that the illness gave the patient. Such ideas have become regarded as naive among psychoanalysts, but in geriatric psychiatry, these mental mechanisms can often be seen at work in the ways that Freud and Adler described.

The symptom is meant to dominate the family. The subconscious motive is that if the parent, usually a widowed mother, is sick enough and demands enough attention, then the children will give up their other responsibilities to attend to her needs. Some of these mothers are insatiable. First of all, they produce symptoms that demand their children's continuous presence, and then use this as a reason for moving into one of their homes. They then find that the daughter or daughter-in-law is not continuously available, and produce further symptoms to ensure their continuous presence. Such parents may eventually "outsmart" themselves, as illustrated by the following case.

> A daughter had hired, out of meager earning, a home aide to sit with her mother while the daughter went out to work. The mother would persuade the aide to make urgent telephone calls to the daughter's workplace, saying that the daughter was immediately needed at home because her mother was ill. The daughter's life became so intolerable that she yielded to pressure from her friends and doctor to put her mother in a nursing home.

Inside the nursing home, the secondary gain is lost, but this does not make the symptoms disappear. The symptoms increase and multiply. In the medically oriented nursing home, they are treated with an ever-increasing variety of medications. Meanwhile the patient becomes older and physically sicker, and more and more incapacitated.

PANIC ATTACKS AND AGORAPHOBIA

Most often with panic attacks and agoraphobia in the elderly, it will be found that the condition has occurred before, in young adult life, and has been misdiagnosed, usually as some physical condition. A typical case is that of an elderly female with a lifelong history of vaguely diagnosed poor physical health who has always avoided going out of the house. On the loss of her husband and other social supports she is admitted to a nursing home. In the nursing home she complains of weakness, dizziness, and palpitations and secludes herself in her room. In the past, females were encouraged to restrict their lives, and could avoid exposing themselves to agoraphobia situations, regarding themselves as frail and fragile. However Luchins and Rose (1989) described three cases in which the onset was in the eighth decade.

Agoraphobia and panic attacks present, even in the young, in a highly somaticized way. The first presentation is often to the cardiologist with complaints of palpitations or to the neurologist with complaints of dizziness and tingling hands and feet, or to the internist with complaints of epigastric discomfort. The somatic nature of these complaints becomes emphasized in the nursing home because they are relayed to the nurse, who then passes them on to the doctor in a summarized form that may not convey the urgency of the anxiety which accompanies them. The result of this is often the prescription of multiple medications.

Psychiatric consultation in a nursing home was requested because of complaints that a patient "carried on in the evenings," with episodes of shouting that disturbed other residents. She had been admitted to the nursing home following hospitalization for a hip fracture.

She described herself as having been "always nervous." She could only stand with support, and required help for most activities of daily living. Her memory was slightly impaired. She knew she was in a nursing home but could not name it.

She said that her main concern was "I'm trying to get out" and expressed discontent at being in a nursing home, and a wish to return home. The predominant mood was one of fear and anxiety. She complained of attacks of shortness of breath and nervousness. These occurred in the evenings and resulted in her crying or calling for help. Her description of these suggested that they were panic attacks. Other organic etiologies were ruled out and she derived considerable benefit from discussion and re-assurance concerning the nature of panic attacks. Literature and in-service education about panic attacks and agoraphobia were provided to the staff members dealing with her.

AGITATION VERSUS ANXIETY

One can imagine intuitively that being demented might create a state of bewilderment and fear of being unable to cope with the world; on the other hand, anxiety is often reduced by alcohol or other drugs that impair awareness. It can be difficult to assess the subjective emotions of the severely demented because their communication is limited, al-though states such as depression have been evaluated with some accu-racy. Patients in the early stages of dementia can tell us if they feel anxiety (Wands et al., 1990), but the diagnosis of anxiety in severely demented patients (Forsell and Winblad, 1997; Folks, 1999b) is prob-lematic. Anxiety in the noncommunicating cannot be assumed on the basis of increased activity and unhappy facial expression alone.

Cohen (1998) has suggested that states labeled as agitation in Alzheimer's disease are manifestations of anxiety. These states are characterized by restlessness, hyperactivity, sweating, and palpita-tions. He has proposed the terms "challenge anxiety," "unfamiliarity anxiety," "unstructure anxiety," and "isolation anxiety" of Alzhei-mer's disease. (See Table 14.1.)

PSYCHOTHERAPY

We are accustomed to thinking of individual psychotherapy as the treatment of choice for the neuroses. Sometimes this resource may be available and useful (Sadavoy and Dorion, 1984) although often it is neither. The provision of psychotherapy to demented patients has even been regarded as a questionable activity (see Chapter 8). The therapist may be suspected of automatically claiming any time spent in the same room with the patient as psychotherapy. The patient may be unaware of receiving any benefit. To avoid questions about moti-vation, it may be best to insist that any classical psychodynamically oriented individual therapy be conducted in a private office away from the nursing home.

TABLE 14.1. Cohen's Classification of Anxiety in Alzheimer's Disease

Type	Precipitants	Nonpharmacological Management
Challenge anxiety	Inability to complete a task, such as answering a question. Analogous to Goldstein's catastrophic reaction	Behavioral distraction. Analogous to handling of child's temper tantrums
Unfamiliarity anxiety	Change in environment, unfamiliar surroundings, different caregivers, or unfamiliar people	
Isolation anxiety	Lack of engagement with environment or people around—analogous to separation anxiety of children	Psychosocial interventions aimed at altering the experience
Unstructure anxiety	Unstructured engagement with surroundings and people	

Source: Cohen, 1998.

In the private office setting, panic attacks and agoraphobia are often treated by behavioral therapy approaches; however, in the institutionalized patient, these can raise the suspicion that the patient is being punished or disciplined. An anxious patient can sometimes be treated with a program of graduated exposure to feared situations and lose the physical symptoms and disabilities, but terms such as "setting limits" and "destimulating" should be avoided.

In spite of these limitations on formal psychotherapy, patients and their families repeatedly express appreciation for time spent talking with friendly and caring staff. One of the major complaints about doctors is that they do not spend enough time talking to patients. Psychopharmacology is sometimes so quick and effective that even psychiatrists may yield to the temptation to dally at the nursing station prescribing, rather than in the patient's room talking.

Controversies and ambiguities will always occur in treatment of these fascinating conditions. Those who manage them must learn to cope with ambiguity and accept the patient's disorder as psychological. Most of the harm is likely to occur from treating the patient rightly for the wrong ailment, rather than by treating incorrectly for the right ailment.

SLEEP DISORDERS

Insomnia is a common complaint of the old. They may sleep less and probably sleep worse. Approximately one-tenth of them take sleeping pills (Bundlie, 1998). Complaints of daytime sleepiness and fatigue are common, and the elderly develop an "early to bed, early to rise" pattern. Total sleep time at night is reduced, although this may be compensated for by daytime naps so that the total time in bed increases. The proportion of sleep that is the lightest kind of sleep (stage 1 sleep) increases. The deeper kinds of sleep (stage 3 sleep and stage 4 sleep, associated with delta waves on the EEG) decrease both absolutely and as a proportion of total sleep. The amount of rapid eye movement (REM) sleep, the kind of sleep in which we dream, decreases absolutely, but remains the same as a proportion of total sleep. In dementia all the sleep changes of aging are increased and REM sleep in particular is diminished (Bundlie, 1998).

In young outpatients, sleep disorders are commonly investigated by such techniques as all night monitoring of the electroencephalograph and eye movements (electronystagmography) but monitoring in nursing home patients is difficult (Waldhorn, 1989).

Being in a nursing home can exacerbate age-related sleep difficulties (Cruise at al., 1999). The normal aging sleep changes are further altered in the nursing home by the organization of day and night activities, changes of shift, prompted voiding regimes for incontinence, times of meals, and schedules of care. Patients' bedtimes tend to be adjusted in a procrustean manner to suit these exigencies.

Daytime naps might be expected to reduce nighttime sleep; and, indeed, many experts in dealing with insomnia recommend that they should be avoided. However, Regenstein and Morris (1987) found that among demented nursing home patients, those who slept most in the day also slept most at night. This might be taken to mean that the elderly nursing home patient need not be deprived of an afternoon nap. Benefits may be found in napping. Some patients become upset if deprived of naps, and the repetitious request to "put me to bed" is often heard in the nursing home. The horizontal position also spreads out weight and, if assumed for less that two hours, may help to prevent the development of pressure sores over the ischial tuberosities.

Insomnia can be a subjective complaint by the patient, and may be a primary concern of the caregivers. Although hypnotics are commonly prescribed in nursing homes, the complaint does not necessarly coincide with the prescription. Cohen and colleagues (1983) studied nondemented nursing home residents and found that many of them did suffer from sleep disorders, as diagnosed by a thirty-minute structured interview. However, these residents with self-reported sleep disorders were not the ones identified by the staff as suffering sleep disturbance, or as needing sleep medications.

ANTIANXIETY MEDICATIONS AND SLEEPING PILLS

Drugs that reduce anxiety and drugs that induce sleep have much in common clinically, biochemically, and in the extent to which the government regulates their use in nursing homes. These multipurpose drugs include the benzodiazepines. Several older drugs such as phenobarbital and other barbiturates, meprobamate, and chloral hydrate (introduced in 1868) that were quite effective are seldom used today, although, as Folks (1999a) points out, it is best to allow elderly patients who think they benefit from these drugs to continue using them.

Clinically, these drugs resemble alcohol in tending to cause addiction, liability to falls, and impairment of memory. The effects on memory often include a slight immediate deleterious effect, a long-term damaging effect on the brain if high dosages are taken, and acute confusion if stopped abruptly after being used for extended periods. Seizures and mental disturbance can occur during withdrawal. They also cause drowsiness, and in some cases, custom alone determines whether a particular drug is regarded as an antianxiety drug or a sleeping pill. Biochemically these similarities in effect are probably because all these substances act on the $GABA_A$ (γ-aminobutyric acid) receptor of the nerve cell.

Most traditional sleeping medications, such as chloral hydrate and barbiturates, have the disadvantages of losing their effect due to tolerance, suppressing REM sleep, and disrupting stage IV sleep (Folks,

1999b). Unsteadiness on their feet the next day is more likely, in theory, with long-acting sedatives such as flurazepam, but short-acting ones, such as triazolam (Halcion) can be just as bad. A patient suffering frequency of urination may want to get up in the night to go to the bathroom and then fall due to grogginess (unless restrained to prevent getting up).

The legal limitations on sedative use in nursing homes have been discussed in Chapter 10. In board and care homes, the HCFA regulations are less onerous, but the absence of registered nursing staff complicates matters. If the staff control medication, then they must either give it on a steady basis or make a decision, which they may not be qualified to make, as to who needs it. One solution is to have patients control their own medication entirely, as they would in entirely independent living situations, but this assumes a capacity for judgment that most do not have.

For Whose Benefit?

As mentioned earlier, being a nuisance to the staff at night, rather than being subjectively tormented by insomnia, is more likely to cause a patient to receive sleeping pills. The fact that nursing home patients often take their sleeping pills early in the evening (Opedal, Schjøtt, and Eide, 1998) may indicate that they are not being allowed to see for themselves if they really are unable to sleep.

Statements by staff that the patient is anxious are sometimes accompanied by, or even preceded by, a request for medication, and it may be necessary to clarify the requestor's priorities. Is the drug for the comfort of the patient or the caregiver? (Not that the latter is a trivial consideration.) On the other hand, denying relief of anxiety because of a wish to avoid running foul of state agencies may not be justified.

The "abuse" of medications in nursing homes can arise from the wishes of patients themselves. Rather than being imposed upon the elderly, the use of sleeping pills and antianxiety drugs can be a mild addictive behavior of their own choice. Currently, the medicines most often craved by patients are the benzodiazepines.

Buspirone

Buspirone (Buspar) is an antianxiety drug which, unlike most others, does not cause drowsiness or addiction. This presumably is because it does not act, as most hypnotic-anxiolytic drugs do, on the $GABA_A$ receptor. The obverse side of its failure to cause drowsiness or addiction is that patients do not experience an immediate sensation of anxiety relief, which may be why it has not achieved the popularity of the benzodiazepines.

Off-Label Drugs

Nursing homes may tend to avoid using specific sleeping medications to evade OBRA restrictions, and thus use such drugs as hydroxyzine (Atarax) and diphenhydramine (Benadryl), which have incidental sedative effects for off-label uses (see Chapter 10). Antidepressants that have sedative effects such as trazodone (Desyrel) and mirtazapine (Remeron) are also used in this way.

Documentation

Although it is tempting to criticize the bureaucratic zeal to multiply paper, the need to document just why a medication is being used can have a salutary effect on prescribing habits. Failure to indicate the rationale for the prescription of a nighttime sedative is frequent. The nursing home staff commonly call the doctor late at night for such orders. This can result in a telephone order being given, which the doctor countersigns at his next visit. At that visit he or she talks to the day staff, not to the ones who asked for the telephone order. Physicians and visiting mental health professionals should make themselves familiar with such matters as when the shifts change and what the staffing ratios are on each shift.

Chapter 15

Wandering, Falls, Physical Restraints, and Loss of Mobility

Wandering, falls, and loss of mobility are closely related. Loss of mobility and wandering might seem to be at opposite ends of a spectrum, but they can be problems in the same patient at the same time. This is because a common reason for use of restraints is to stop the wobbly from wandering and falling. Problems in restraint removal center around very demented patients whom the staff is afraid might fall (Sullivan-Marx et al., 1999). We have all seen the patients who insist on getting up and walking but fall when they do so (unless adequate help is available to support them). Restraints prevent falls to a certain extent by preventing the patient from getting up in the first place, but may not actually reduce the number of injuries (Tideiksaar, 1998). One reason for this is the "use it or lose it" effect. The muscles of the nonambulant patients can become so weak that when they are allowed to get up their muscles will not support them.

WANDERING

Wandering is a symptom especially difficult to deal with in nursing homes and, in fact, nursing homes that do not have locking doors may not accept severe wanderers as patients.

All wanderers are not alike, and mild wanderers may be manageable in a nursing home. The definition of a mild wanderer is not exact. Some attempt can be made to classify wanderers, although little literature or experimental work on this exists (Klein et al., 1999) (see Table 15.1).

TABLE 15.1. Types of Wandering

Type	Causes	Distance traveled	Complications	Management
Aimless	Severe dementia with disorientation. Delirium. Visual impairment. Strange surroundings.	Very short. Seldom outside building.	Falls. Use of restraints. Intruding into space of others	Redirection. Close supervision. Treatment of cause of delirium. Bright lights. Ophthalmic assessment. Reorientation.
Insistent	Mild dementia (may be more common in Pick's disease). Delusions and hallucinations. Reduplicative paramnesia.	Walking distance. Often insist on going outside.	Violence when prevented. Exposure. Wandering into traffic.	Door latches requiring cognitive skill to open. Shadowing and following. Do not chase on foot. Antipsychotic medication.
Fugues	Slight dementia. Paranoid disorder.	May travel hundreds of miles using public transport or driving.	May drive automobile and get into accidents. Distress to caregivers and family. May become permanently missing.	Attached ID such as name bracelets. Transponder devices. Prevention of access to automobiles.

Wandering may be called mild if the distance traveled is short, and if the wanderer is easily turned back by simple redirecting. Wandering is more severe when the wanderer insists on going out and violently refuses to be returned home. Such wandering can usually be easily circumvented in an institution by means of electronic and architectural devices but can give rise to a physical dispute when the patient is at home.

A demented but able-bodied man insisted on walking outside at night and would threaten violence if prevented. Family members arranged to follow him by car. When he appeared exhausted, they stopped and offered him a ride. He would then come quietly home.

A rather separate category of elaborate fugues exists. These patients travel great distances in an apparently purposeful way, especially if provided with cash.

A seventy-year-old man was seen because of memory loss. He was, when questioned, unable to state his age, the date, or to identify his family members by name. However, he subsequently made his way over fifty miles to Kennedy Airport, and traveled to Ireland, where he was found wandering and disoriented.

The severe types of wandering usually occur in the middle stages of dementia. The symptom tragically cures itself as the dementia gets worse, because extremely severe dementia produces immobility.

The complications of wandering, accidents, and immobility can be divided into their effects on the staff, and their effects on the patients. The adverse psychological effects on nursing home staff of patients' wandering can be quite severe. Fears arise of dangerous places into which they might intrude. Sometimes kitchens are mentioned, and sometimes other residents' rooms. If the patient leaves the building, anxiety is profound. Staff may be taken off the floors to go outside to look for the patient.

The actual adverse effects on the patients are less evident, and it is most unusual to find that they are any worse for wear when they return. No statistical evidence suggests that they are especially liable to accidents or injury. In very cold climates they are vulnerable to hypothermia.

In the board and care homes, wandering is accepted more casually, and treated in much the same way as when it occurs in the general population. After a resident has been missing for a day, he or she may be reported to the police as missing. The willingness of the police to treat the case as a missing person varies with jurisdictions. The amount of hue and cry may depend on whether the rent has been paid.

Causes

The paradox that wandering and loss of mobility have much in common persists in regard to their causes. The same factors that cause wandering may also cause accidents that lead to immobility, or the imposition of restraints, which obviously cause immobility.

Confusion

Disorientation can be a symptom of dementia, and naturally, may give rise to wandering. Sleeping pills and benzodiazepines can produce a disoriented hyperactive state akin to that sometimes produced by alcohol and thus cause wandering.

Delusions

Delusions may give rise to elaborate fugues.

> A paranoid woman in an adult home regularly makes visits to a famous restaurant in New York that she claims to own. She makes the trip by bus and subway. The management usually sends her back by car at their expense.

Visual Impairment

Blindness is a common cause of wandering into other residents' rooms.

Neurological Illness

Akathisia is a cause of restless pacing with inability to get comfortable in one position. It may be due to Parkinson's disease or to drug-induced parkinsonism. Complex partial seizures can manifest themselves as wandering.

Environment

Sometimes a new environment is more disorienting and causes increased wandering, for example, in attempts to find the bathroom. On the other hand, changes of environment can also reduce wandering. Architectural features can be important; single-story buildings with several exits are more difficult to police. A nursing home located in a mild climate, with large grounds in an area remote from busy traffic is better able to cope with wanderers.

Case Mix

A patient mix that includes bedridden patients along with those who have no physical illness below the neck increases the likelihood of wandering and of loss of mobility. The bedridden will have bed-sores and other ailments, which necessitate the staff being at their bedside, especially the skilled nursing staff. This will make it difficult to keep the fully mobile residents within sight. The skilled nursing activity becomes focused on the hands-on technical procedures rather than helping the fully ambulant become involved in psychosocial treatments; and the ambulant are left to their own devices, if they are allowed to be ambulant at all.

Prevention and Management

A nursing home must first recognize its limitations in dealing with wandering. Screening out potential wanderers is one way to do this. OBRA '87 was geared toward giving nursing home residents greater freedom from sedative drugs and physical restraints. The framers of the act seemed to be under the impression that fully mobile patients with dementia can safely be handled in nursing homes, but nursing homes often find it especially difficult to handle able-bodied patients with purely behavioral disturbances. The fact that the behavioral disturbances are due to dementia does not ease the situation. Certainly a wandering problem should be anticipated when the demented are considered for admission. When a potential wanderer is admitted, it should be made clear to all concerned that the home is not locked and is not a secure facility. It may be best to have this statement in writing, signed by those responsible for the placement. However, this is rather legalistic and defensive, and should be supplemented by programs that make families aware of the different ways of dealing with wandering.

Some of the architectural modifications possible for dementia units have been described. They include measures (that must comply with fire regulations) to make it more complicated to open doors. The simplest such device consists of an arrangement of two buttons that must be pressed in sequence to open a door, thus making it inaccessible to the severely demented. Local chapters of the Alzheimer's Disease Association have other recommendations.

Many electronic gadgets are now on the market. In general, the objections to these have been expense and the difficulty of persuading patients to keep them on. Some operate like the tags in department stores that sound an alarm at the exit door when a shoplifter walks out with a stolen item. Transponders that actually locate the wanderer are available. A loud alarm when an exit door is opened will deter many.

When patients have left the building, a rehearsed and preplanned drill should be instituted for returning them. It is better to use law enforcement officers to retrieve patients than to require badly needed staff from the home to chase them. Chasing can be dangerous and may cause the pursued to run into traffic.

The major weapon for dealing with wandering, falls, accidents, and immobility is education. The more everyone knows about these situations, the less dangerous they will be.

FALLS

Falls are responsible for one-fourth of the admissions to nursing homes (Tinetti and Williams, 1997). Falls can be classified in various ways.

Studies consistently show distinctions between the single-time faller and the multiple faller. The single-time fallers, whether or not they suffer fractures, are not well distinguished from the general population. Multiple fallers are demented but ambulant, have poor vision, and are on psychotropics. A study by Tideiksaar (1986) well demarcates the single-time fallers from the multiple fallers (see Table 15.2).

The presence of injury or fractures is another distinction between types of falls. Serious falls are more common among multiple fallers. Those who get injured are more independent and less depressed (Tinetti, 1987).

TABLE 15.2. Elderly Fallers

Single-time fallers	Similar to general population.	Less likely to suffer fracture or injury.
Multiple fallers	Demented but ambulant. Psychotropic medication. Poor vision.	Frequent injury and fracture.

Source: Tideiksaar, 1986.

Fall Predictors

In a study by Brody and colleagues (1984) of institutionalized elderly women with Alzheimer's disease, those who fell were not so much the inactive or the very active, but those who had been active and whose vigor had declined. It seemed that there was a wish to retain full mobility with a failure to realize limitations. Robbins and colleagues (1989) give multiple medications, hip weakness, and poor balance as the strongest fall predictors. Visual impairment predicted strongly in Tideiksaar's study. The influence of medication is discussed further later on.

Osteoporosis

Among fractures is a group related to osteoporosis, which are liable to occur with minimal injury. The osteoporosis-related fractures (neck of femur, wrist, and compression fracture of spine) are generally more common among women, but after men have been in a nursing home for many years, their incidence rises as well (Rudman and Rudman, 1989).

Falls and Medication

Many elderly people fall regardless of drugs. The consensus of the literature and clinical experience is that those taking psychotropic medications are more liable to fall but the numbers are difficult to reliably crunch (Leipzig, Cummings, and Tinetti, 1999) and it cannot be assumed that most falls are medication related. One-third of all those in the community over seventy-five years old fall every year, most of them more than once (Tinetti, Speechley, and Ginter, 1988).

Even the new and improved antidepressants are associated with falls, especially if they are used for behavior control in the demented rather than for definite depression (Thapa et al., 1998). Caramel et al. (1998) found that very old community-living patients in Holland were four times more likely to fall when taking long-acting benzodiazepines than those taking the short-acting medication. Short-acting benzodiazepines used as sleeping pills produce a vulnerable interval between taking the medication and getting into bed. Supervision at this time might be expected to reduce the risk (although this has not been statistically proven).

The relationship between medication and other fall prediction factors is complex. In a long-term facility, Granek and colleagues (1987) found that the two diagnoses and the two groups of drugs most frequently associated with falling were osteoarthritis and depression and antidepressants and hypnotics. Taking three or more drugs was especially likely to be associated with falling, the most potent combination in this respect being diuretic + NSAID + hypnotic. They point out that the side effects of NSAIDs (nonsteroidal antiinflammatory drugs) can include confusion, mood changes, and dizziness.

Complications

The adverse effects of accidents are also most severe upon the staff. Accidents cause time-consuming paperwork, fear of litigation, and fear of adverse comments by state inspectors.

Regarding adverse effects on the patient, the kind of accident that occurs in a nursing home is usually never fatal. Pain and the need for a visit to the hospital may be experienced. The major adverse consequence, however, is loss of mobility, and this must be taken into account in attempts to settle the argument about the patients who are being restrained from walking, because of fears that their gait may cause a fall.

PHYSICAL RESTRAINTS

The chances of an inmate in an institution being restrained vary from time to time and place to place. Nursing home residents used to be tied up or caged in for much of their lives (Evans and Strumpf, 1989). The acute care general hospitals also had a bad track record regarding restraints, and patients on acute medical and surgical floors have been restrained with greater impunity to the staff than those on psychiatric floors. The Joint Committee on Accreditation of Health Care Organizations, which set standards in 1997, now promises to raise them to the standards demanded of jails and state psychiatric hospitals. In the board and care homes and assisted living accommodations, the use of restraints is seldom an issue. It seems to be assumed (and is sometimes legally mandated) that residents have the same rights to be free as do other adult Americans.

The use of restraints varies considerably from state to state (Braun, 1999). It is lowest in Iowa and highest in Alaska. No empirical studies of the reasons for this have been undertaken. States with high retraint use tend to have low rates of nursing home institutionalization. This could reflect that in these states nursing home residents are sicker or more behaviorally disturbed. Patients who mouth off and become disliked by the staff are likely to find themselves physically restrained for longer times (Schnelle, Simmons, and Ory, 1992).

Legal Restraints on Restraints

In the five years following OBRA '87, the use of restraints in nursing homes declined by half (Grossberg, 1993). Federal law now states that a nursing home resident "has the right to be free from any physical restraints imposed or psychoactive drug administered for purposes of discipline or convenience, and not required to treat the resident's medical symptoms" (Braun, 1999, p. 2).

HCFA Interpretive Guidelines for surveyors defined a physical restraint as "any manual method or physical or mechanical device, material or equipment attached or adjacent to the resident's body that the resident cannot move easily which restricts freedom of movement or normal access to one's body" (Braun, 1999, p. 2). Restraints cannot be ordered as needed ("PRN"). The physician must justify use and alternatives must be considered. Restrained residents are to be released, exercised, and repositioned every two hours.

In order to claim that a device is applied to "treat the resident's medical condition," it will probably need to qualify as a safety device or a mechanical support, rather than as a restraint. If such a distinction can indeed be made, then a mechanical support must be used on a patient who does not have the mobility to resist it. For example, a chair designed to support a quadriplegic in an upright sitting position without falling over would be a mechanical support, but a chair designed to frustrate its occupant's deliberate attempts to get out is a retraint. Certain patients slide out of chairs to the floor if left unsupported and find this happening to them involuntarily. A device to prevent this justifies the term "mechanical support."

One criterion is whether the restraint is under the control of the person it is imposed upon. A car seatbelt, which we can take on and off ourselves, is not a restraint. Some who are wheelchair bound are liable to fall forward out of their chairs by pulling themselves up to a table (Gold, Gordon, and Silber, 1988). If a belt is needed to prevent such a contingency, then to be termed a safety device and not a restraint, it must be capable of being unfastened by its wearer. A complicated door fastening, which can be opened by the nondemented but not by the demented, is not a restraint.

The Antirestraint Movement

These restraint reductions would perhaps have come about even without OBRA. One factor has been an increase in the sophistication and availability of electronic devices. Bed alarms of several kinds can now warn if a patient is climbing out of bed or is wandering. It is also possible that increased use of mental health experts has helped to make retraints regarded as old-fashioned and cruel. Arguments about restraint use resemble those concerning hitting children. The liberal modern tendency is to avoid it. The side that sees itself as enlightened and progressive has a visceral dislike of the practice, claims to have scientific evidence against it, and believes it can and should be abolished. The other side invokes tradition and common sense, and believes it to be safe and sometimes necessary. Assessment of the evidence is colored by prejudice.

The Kendal Corporation is a nonprofit organization devoted to ending restraint use in nursing homes. It provides useful literature, including a newsletter titled "Unbind the Elderly" (PO Box 100, Kennett Square, PA 19348), a Web site <www.ute.kendal.org>, and audiovisual material.

Types of Restraints

Geri-chairs, vest restraints, and side rails are among the most common restraining devices used in nursing homes.

Geri-chair is a trademark name for what is less commonly, but more properly, called an institutional chair. The essential feature is that it can be wheeled by an attendant, but not self-propelled by the patient. Sometimes a capacity for restraint is added by a kind of feeding tray that fits across the front, or by a device that converts it into a lay-back chair. There are small wheels on casters. The Geri-chair may be used as a battering ram by the agitated patient. Its main role in increasing violence, however, is simply that it takes up space. Two patients in Geri-chairs are more likely to encounter each other than two who are walking. The very determined patients will get themselves around even in a Geri-chair, by attaching themselves to railings, furniture, or other patients. Accidents can then result from the chair capsizing together with its occupant. Patients also get out of them by sliding downward and forward. This tendency is sometimes prevented by the lay-back device or by a pelvic restraint.

Geri-chairs with feeding trays are probably a restraint under the federal regulations, which define the restraint as any device for preventing mobility that the patient cannot remove easily which restricts freedom of movement or normal access to one's body. Some state mental health departments seem to exempt the Geri-chair by defining a restraint only as a device that prevents free movement of the arms and legs, and thus allow them to be used in psychiatric units.

"Posey" refers to JT Posey and Co., who make a line of soft inconspicuous restrains. The commonly used "soft Posey vest restraint" is a garment that can be fastened at the back to a chair, so as to prevent the sitter from getting up. Sometimes the patient gets up in spite of it by lifting up the chair, and this can cause nasty accidents.

Side rails are of various kinds. They can be safe if the patient is under continuous observation in an intensive care unit or during recovery from anesthesia, but can undoubtedly cause accidents, mainly because patients try to climb over them (Tideiksaar and Osterwell, 1989). It is still undecided whether side rails legally constitute restraints (Plichta, 1998). They can harm patients in all sorts of ways (Miles and Parker, 1998). I have known a patient to suffer a compound fracture of the tibia by becoming tangled in the side rails and falling from the bed. Half rails, which do not go down to the bottom of the bed, are safer. If the patient is liable to roll out of bed, it is safer still to put the mattress on the floor.

Do Restraints Prevent Accidents?

A common rationale is that the patient may fall if not restrained and that the staff will be blamed for this, whereas they are not to be blamed for injuries or illness due to the restraints. Other reasons cited by Evans and Strumpf (1989) as being given for applying restraints are wandering, pulling out tubes, agitation, confusion, "to assure good body alignment," administrative pressure, and insufficient staffing. Although the evidence is conflicting, it is clear that restraints are not a panacea for preventing falls (Braun, 1999). Probably two reasons account for this failure. One is that the restraints may be used as a substitute for observation, with unobserved patients falling while restrained. Another is that the restraints cause the patients' gait to become less steady when they are allowed to walk, perhaps because of disuse muscle atrophy or postural hypotension. Falls while in restraints are most likely to occur in the agitated patient who is resisting the restraint and attempting to escape from it.

Do Restraints Prevent Lawsuits?

Many nursing home staff believe that they may be sued because a patient falls as a result of not being restrained. In the frequently quoted case in which a patient wandered off into traffic and was killed by a car driven by his daughter, the point at issue was not that he should have been locked up but that no one noticed he was gone from the nursing home (Tammalleo, 1988). Two cases in which unrestrained patients fell that most closely resemble this scenario (*Swain v. Lean-Care Rest Home* in North Carolina and *Hubby v. South Alabama Nursing Home* cited by Kapp, 1999) were decided on the basis of whether supervision was adequate. Several legal decisions suggest that restraints can generate litigation rather than protect against it (the three Louisiana cases of *Booty v. Kenwood Nursing Home,* 1985; *Field v. Senior Citizen Center,* 1988; and *McGillivray Ray v. Rapids Iberia Management Enterprises,* 1986; and also the Alabama case of *Ruby Davis v. Mantras Bay Care Center,* 1989, also cited in Kapp, 1999).

Adverse Consequences of Restraints

Much of our knowledge of the risk/benefits ratio of restraints is impressionistic and reflects individual prejudice for or against restraints. Studies in hospitalized patients do suggest a direct effect of restraints in causing death (Frengley and Mion, 1986). Possible adverse consequences of restraints include increased severity of injury due to falls that do occur (e.g., from climbing over side rails or tipping over chairs), loss of functional capacity, aspiration pneumonia, decubitus ulcers, osteoporosis, increased agitation, anger, demoralization, and humiliation. In practice, more depends on staff attitudes than what statistics show.

Restraint-Free Units

Successful demonstration of a restraint-free unit is needed to convince the skeptics. Coercion of staff cannot be used to start such a unit. Each nursing home will have some staff members who firmly believe that patients cannot be safely treated without using restraints and others with different viewpoints. When restrainers are mixed with libertarians the restrainers always win. There will be a point at which, regardless of all exhortation from authority, a restrainer will put a patient in restraints and announce that the measure was absolutely necessary "for the patient's safety."

A restraint-free unit must be staffed by convinced libertarians. The first step is to identify these individuals by means of surveys and discussions. They are then recruited to staff the restraint-free unit. Once the unit is set up, it will speak for itself.

LOSS OF MOBILITY

In comparison to falls and wandering, immobility does not cause as much psychological upset to the staff, and they may not even regard it as a problem (Selikson, Damus, and Hammerman, 1988). The Minimum Data Set, however, will pick up loss of mobility as a trigger for a Resident Assessment Protocol (see Chapter 2) and thus focus attention on it. In addition to the MDS, different disciplines, such as physiotherapy, have devised their own scales for measuring loss of mobility.

Adverse Effects and Causes

Immobility results in adverse physical effects on the patient that are frequently fatal. The immobile patients develop muscle atrophy and fixed contractures of the limbs. They become incontinent of urine and feces and prone to infections and bedsores, from which they eventually die.

Policy

Immobility can result from policies of state reimbursement or administration. Patients who go out overnight to stay with families, go away on vacations, or go shopping may have their Medicaid funds cut off. Time spent on such activities is considered to be time in which the patient does not need skilled nursing care. The need to be the recipient of skilled nursing care is financially and legally incumbent on every nursing home resident. Being strapped into a chair assists this because, if the beneficiary of this treatment protests too vigorously, the protests can be quelled by medication, and the dispensing and careful recording of medication doses is undoubtedly a skilled nursing function.

Age and Nonpsychiatric Illness

Age itself causes loss of muscle mass and ability to exercise vigorously. Many systemic medical conditions, such as congestive heart failure and fever, are accompanied by asthenia. The treating of medical conditions by bed rest is still in vogue to some extent.

Fractures

Loss of mobility is especially liable to follow fractures. Many demented nursing home patients fail to walk again after surgery for a hip fracture. It has even been suggested (Lyon and Nevins, 1984) that, from the rehabilitation point of view, it is not worth operating on the demented elderly nursing home patient with a hip fracture (although the operation may also have the function of relieving pain). Certainly, the management of hip fractures is not just a matter of pinning the broken ends of the bone together; complex psychosocial factors are involved (Nickens, 1983).

Tubes

If tubes of any kind have been inserted into any orifice to improve the patient's condition, then the care and maintenance of these tubes becomes a matter of priority, which demands skilled nursing care and preempts any other aspect of care. The fully mobile patient may pull out these life-sustaining tubes. The common response to this is to tie the patient's wrists.

Psychiatric Conditions

Depression is the most likely psychiatric condition to reduce mobility. The effects of dementia are complex. Many demented patients show increased motor activity and, as has been described, this can result in use of medication and other measures to slow them down. The end stages of demented illness are often marked by loss of all capacity for control of motor function. The patient literally forgets how to walk.

It must also be said that, even in the absence of specific psychiatric illness, the patients themselves sometimes resist mobilization. Pawlson, Goodwin, and Keith (1986) studied nursing home residents who had taken to using wheelchairs although they were medically able to walk. Their spontaneously expressed reasons for using the wheelchairs were vague and expressed as some kind of general physical impairment, but when specifically asked, most of them agreed that fear of falling was a reason for using the chairs. They also used the chairs to get into strategic attention-getting situations. Officially designated seating areas for patients are often in lounges or recreation areas, but many like to congregate in corridors or close to the nursing station.

These authors found that the use of the wheelchair often coincided with admission to the nursing home. They suggest that this may relate to the nursing home as being an environment in which wheelchairs are easy to obtain and use. The elderly person in his or her own home has often become accustomed to getting around by hanging onto the furniture, and stairs, steps, and narrow doorways may have impeded wheelchair use.

It will sometimes seem that the old are poorly motivated toward rehabilitation and desire only rest and surcease. These poorly motivated elderly patients can easily be excluded from rehabilitation programs (Hesse and Campion, 1983), but such exclusion may eventually reduce their total well-being.

Chapter 16

Violence

Nursing home residents can be quite violent, and violence looms surprisingly large in nursing homes. Geriatric psychiatrists find that a high proportion of their referrals result from instances of aggression and violence (Shah, 1993). Among psychogeriatric patients, aggressive behavior increases with age and with severity of dementia (Nilsson, Palmstierna, and Wisted, 1988; Tsai et al., 1996; Ryden, 1988). The association of violence with the male sex persists in old age.

The board and care homes contain potentially explosive mixtures of mental illness, alcoholism, and drug addiction. In New York State adult homes, half the residents are former psychiatric hospital patients and one-third of all residents are over sixty-five (Mesnikoff and Wilder, 1983). This patient mix contains a high potential for violence. I encounter homicide or rape in these places once or twice a year.

The possibility of violence by the staff exists, but the slightest question of violence by staff against patients is always rigorously investigated by state authorities (whereas violence by patients against staff is governmentally ignored). These inquisitions can be demoralizing for staff who find themselves subjected daily to insults and violence by those they tend. Considerable moral support and mutual encouragement may be needed.

RISK FACTORS

Psychiatric Illness

Dementia and Delirium

Among psychiatric diagnoses, the one most commonly associated with violence in the elderly is dementia (Burns, Jacoby, and Levy, 1990), which cannot always be readily distinguished in acute situa-

tions from delirium. On standardized ward behavior rating scales, Alzheimer patients score quite high for aggression, as compared to those
with nondementing mental disorders. Their episodes of violence tend
to be brief, without a sustained attack on one person, which limits the
damage they do. Their actual physical damage is further limited by
their age and weakness and physical incapacity. The feebleness of the
attacks by the demented may be counterbalanced by the fact that, in a
nursing home, other residents are also feeble and cannot defend
themselves. The vulnerability of the disabled does not, in and of itself, cause violence. It magnifies the effect of violence. When a frail
osteoporotic woman is pushed in a mild way, she may fall and fracture her hip.

Drugs and Alcohol

Psychiatric disorders that are not age-specific must also be considered, especially among the relatively young populations of the board
and care homes where alcohol and "crack" cocaine are common.
Within the skilled nursing facilities, the benzodiazepines can produce
an effect similar to alcohol. For example, if benzodiazepines are
given in large enough doses they may quiet a violent person and send
him or her off to sleep, but if an intermediate dose is given, a drunken
belligerence may result.

Personality Disorders

The number of violent criminals who survive to nursing home age
is reduced by homicide, suicide, and by drug, tobacco, and alcohol
use. However, thirty thousand inmates of state and federal prisons are
over the age of fifty-five (Butterfield, 1997). Sometimes patients who
have antisocial personalities and previous criminal histories find their
way into nursing homes.

Paranoia and Delusions

Paranoia and delusions can be associated with sustained and dangerous violence, and the likelihood of violence in Alzheimer patients
is increased by the concurrence of delusions (Gormley, Rizwan, and
Lovestone, 1998). An increasing population consists of patients with

a previous history of functional psychosis, usually schizophrenia, who have been released from state hospitals to roam the streets (Isaac and Armat, 1990) or enter board and care homes, and who then fail to take their medication (Butterfield, 1998). Failure to take medication often precedes violence in schizophrenics. These patients are mostly the "young old" in their sixties and early seventies. They are more able-bodied than the demented and can inflict more damage.

Mania

Mania is unusual in the very old but may occur, and is easily mistaken for an agitated state when the patient has a background of pre-existing cognitive impairment (Habib, Birkett, and Devanand, 1998).

> A seventy-year-old man began taking off for long drives at high speed. He caused multiple car crashes, was admitted to hospital for treatment of his injuries, and then transferred to a nursing home. He became disruptive and resistant to care. On psychiatric consultation he was found to be manic. Further history taking revealed a history of several previous bouts of hyperactivity and bizarre behavior.

Depression

Depression in old age commonly presents with somatic symptoms or psychomotor retardation but may eventuate in a suicide/homicide based on delusions. This has not been recorded inside a nursing home, but may be precipitated by the fear of being "put in a home."

> An eighty-year-old man with severe depression but in good physical health became convinced that he and his wife were incurably ill and had lost all their money. He shot and killed her to put her out of her misery and then called the police.

Lyketsos and colleagues (1999) found that among demented patients the presence of depression, rather than delusions and hallucinations, predicted violence. Negative emotions can be difficult to disentangle, and a morose unsmiling individual might be perceived as depressed.

Stroke

Violence is sometimes associated with stroke. Aggression ranks after depression and memory loss among mental changes causing concern to caregivers of stroke victims (Hanger and Mulley, 1993).

> An ambulant demented patient who had had a stroke was discharged from a VA hospital on the grounds that he did not require active medical treatment. He was refused psychiatric hospital care because he was demented and was placed in a nursing home. He walked out of the facility and went home and killed his wife.

Isaacs, Neville, and Rushford (1976) found that among thirty-five stroke patients studied, three showed the pattern of "aggression," with verbal and sometimes physical hostility, usually directed against the spouse. There were ten who showed the pattern of "frustration," with excessive irritability or reluctance to cooperate. Goldstein's (1952) catastrophic reaction consists of sudden emotional outbursts when the patients are not able to fulfill a task set before them.

CLASSIFICATION

Although it is not supported by statistical analysis, clinical experience suggests that geriatric violence can usefully be classified into the following broad categories: aggressive agitation; escalation of nonviolent agitated behavior; acting upon delusions; spousal abuse; resistance to care; fugues and wandering; and sexual assaults. Each of these categories may require either emergency interventions or long-term treatment (see Table 16.1).

Escalation of Nonviolent Agitated Behavior

Behaviors can be antisocial without being violent. In dealing with these, it is often useful to consider the option of tolerating the nonviolent behavior. This type of problem most commonly occurs in an institutional setting in which there is low tolerance for eccentricity.

A patient in an acute care general hospital walked into a nursing station. When he was asked to leave he lay on the floor and refused to move. Security guards were called. They attempted to lift him and he punched and kicked them. Later he was transferred to a nursing home. When he walked into the nursing station there, he was invited to sit down and remained there quietly without causing any trouble.

These nonviolent behaviors may also anger other patients. Some of the demented paw and maul at passersby or intrude into their space in a way that can provoke violence. Obscenities and ethnic slurs from noisy individuals are especially liable to incite violence.

Acting Upon Delusions

When a patient suffers delusions, the violence is more likely to be sustained and organized and the danger of homicide is greater. Guns or knives may be involved (Green and Kellerman, 1996; Petrie, Lawson, and Hollender, 1982), although the nursing home is normally able to prevent access to these.

Identification of the content of the delusions is important in planning management strategies. For example, if the behavior is justified in the patient's mind as a response to imagined persecution, then protection and reassurance can be offered and nonviolent precautions suggested. Treatment of the underlying psychosis by antipsychotic medication is especially likely to help.

Fugues and Wandering

As described in Chapter 15, episodes of fugues and wandering are not intrinsically violent but in some cases, the patient, usually demented or delirious, will insist on going out late at night or in inclement weather. A physical dispute may arise when attempts are made to stop the patient. Wanderers sometimes endanger themselves or others by wandering into traffic, although the demented elderly have a remarkable tendency to stay on sidewalks.

TABLE 16.1. Typology of Psychogeriatric Violence

	Special Diagnostic Points	Special Points in Management
Aggressive agitation	dementia, delirium, mania, physical pain	physical danger not as great because nondirected and often concurrent medical problems and immobility, special need to look for medical causes.
Escalation of nonviolent agitated behavior	dementia, environmental factors	identify circumstances, discuss with staff, avoid unnecessary interventions, do not try to protect property
Acting upon delusions	paranoid disorders, schizophrenia	identify delusions, treatment of psychosis
Spousal abuse	personality disorders, alcohol, cultural factors	high homicide risk
Resistance to care	dementia, physical pain, cultural factors	start care with extra staff, modify medical regime
Fugues and wandering	dementia	use of ID bracelets, electronic devices, head off rather than chase, offer ride home, maintain distance
Sexual assaults	dementia, disinhibition due to drugs/alcohol, localized brain damage	identify victims, discuss with community

Resistance to Care

Situations in which the patients are touched or moved commonly give rise to violence. A prime example is when they are being given morning care, such as washing or changing. Violence directed against staff may also occur when the residents are touched in an attempt to stop a nonviolent antisocial behavior, such as walking into a restricted area, or sitting on the floor, or not going to bed at night, or hawking and retching on the floor.

Defending Turf

Territoriality is at the root of much violence. A frequent victim is a roommate. Some of this is accompanied by delusions, such as accusations of stealing, but a common occurrence is to push or punch at anyone who gets too near.

Violence initiated by contact with other patients often involves wheelchairs. Among their other dangers, these contrivances take up considerable space. Quite often, another patient is bumped, whether ambulant or in another wheelchair, who then responds with violence. This territory factor can sometimes act to make the feeble elderly patients in the nursing home paradoxically more dangerously violent than the younger patients in the board and care homes. The latter can walk away from trouble. On occasion, the police are called to deal with a violent dispute, and by the time they arrive, the parties have left the building or retreated to their rooms.

Rating scales such as Patel and Hope's (1992) Rating Scale for Aggressive Behavior in the Elderly (RAGE), and the Overt Aggression Scale (OAS) of Yudofsky, Silver, and Hales (1990), may be useful not only in research but in clinical practice for assessment of the efficacy of intervention over an extended period of time.

A seventy-five-year-old patient had been a state hospital patient for most of his life with an intractable problem of random violence. His communication was so limited that a precise diagnosis could not be established. His records over the years showed the use of twenty medications, including antipsychotics, mood stabilizers, and anticonvulsants, as well as use of ECT (electroconvulsive therapy) and other modalities. The staff varied in their accounts of the effectiveness of these, and some said that no medication did any good. Following treatment team and family discussions, rating scales were recorded at regular intervals, including drug holidays over a year until all involved agreed on an optimal drug and management regime.

MANAGEMENT

Dealing with physical aggression within an institution should begin with an analysis of the circumstances in which it occurs. This may be helped by familiarity with applied behavior analysis (Burke and Wesolowski, 1988; Burke and Lewis, 1986). Tact is necessary in conducting this analysis to avoid a purported search for justification, blaming the victim, or finding fault with the caregivers. Reluctance to look for patterns may suggest a resentment of being required to deal with such patients at all. This should be explored and discussed. Those involved will tend to say initially that no pattern is evident, and that the perpetrator can be violent at any time and every day.

A seventy-year-old resident in an adult home had previously been a homeless alcoholic. He was quarrelsome and suspicious but not clinically paranoid. He used a walking cane both for ambulation and as a weapon whenever he was annoyed. Medical examination revealed no disability necessitating a walking aid. Physiotherapy consultation and gait training was requested. It was established that he had a stable gait without need for aid. Deprived of his weapon, he limited his aggression to verbal abuse.

In general, the principle should be to remove the victim from the aggressor, rather than the aggressor from the victim. This is especially true in geriatric psychiatry because elderly aggressors are often feeble or confused and will fail to pursue their victim.

I was called late at night to an adult home where an elderly resident with a previous diagnosis of schizophrenia, recently refusing antipsychotic medications, was running around a common recreation area breaking chairs and threatening staff and other residents. When I got there he had retreated to his room. The staff agreed that it would be easier to leave him alone than attempt forcible hospitalization and medication. In the morning, he was calm and agreed to take his antipsychotic medications again. There were no further incidents.

It may be possible to work with administrators to control the patient mix and decide who gets admitted. A roommate is a likely violence victim and, when possible, high-risk patients should not share rooms. Care must be taken in choosing roommates. If possible, the violent patient should be given a single room. Two beds in a triple room may be better than a standard double room. Some areas, such as corridors, need special attention to ensure supervision of contacts between high-risk patients. Keeping distance between patients must be kept in mind when arranging group activities.

Not having the violent patient in the nursing home in the first place is, perhaps, nihilistic, but can be the most practical measure. Certainly those in charge of admissions should be aware of the possibility that the patient is violent and look for danger signals (such as refusal of a previous nursing home to take the patient back). Talking to previous caregivers is useful. If obstacles are placed in the way of this, then suspicion should be aroused.

Violence associated with schizophrenia, mania, and sociopathic personality disorder is seldom manageable in a nursing home. An attempt should be made to move the patient to a secure facility, but this may be difficult to accomplish. The family may resist transfer to a mental hospital because this is felt to be stigmatizing, or because they are afraid (often with good cause) that the mental hospital will discharge the patient and the home will refuse to take the patient back.

The case mix must be looked at from time to time for its violence potential. If possible, the able-bodied demented should be separated from the vulnerable feeble.

The general principle always should be to leave space. Empty space is the most effective straitjacket. There should be a cushion of air around the violent patients, and plenty of room for them to move around. Getting them outdoors may be best.

If violence is directed against staff when the resident is touched in the course of attempting to stop a nonviolent agitated behavior, then ways of dealing with this without touching the patient can be explored. Tolerating some of these nonviolent behaviors may be the best policy.

Resistance during morning care is common. There can be punching, kicking, biting, and scratching. Sometimes this will be with one aide but not with another. Sometimes feelings of personal modesty are involved. It may be suggested that morning care should be initiated with two or three aides present. One of them can serve as bodyguard, protecting the other from blows or punches. It may be objected that there is not enough staff for this, to which there are two rejoinders. The first is that the extra aide is mostly only needed at the beginning of care; once the process is under way it will normally be safe for the second to leave. The second is that this is more economical of staff time than the opposite procedure of initiating care with one aide present and then the aide having to go off and look for someone to help because he or she cannot manage alone.

In Goldstein's catastrophic reaction, the main principle of management is to identify the tasks that cause frustration, and to try to arrange a lifestyle and degree of assistance with activities with communication and activities of daily living that can avert provocation. The services of an occupational therapist can be especially useful in this. A physiotherapist and speech pathologist should also, if possible, take part in formulating a treatment plan.

MEDICATIONS

The efficacy of neuroleptic drugs in treating certain kinds of psychosis is beyond reasonable doubt. In a meta-analysis of trials of antipsychotic drugs in dementia, it was found that conditions of agitation and uncooperativeness tended to improve in most studies, and that conditions of combativeness, assaultiveness, and hostility improved in several double-blind placebo-controlled trials (Schneider, Pollock, and Lyness, 1990).

Nevertheless, there is no drug with an FDA approval for use in treatment of violence. The use of drugs to control violent behavior is often empirical, even if theoretically linked to concepts that the behavior is a manifestation of psychosis, epilepsy, mood disorder, or attention deficit disorder. Attempts have been made to provide a rationale for particular drugs in terms of their action on neurotransmitters (Garner and Garrett, 1997; Mintzer, Hoernig, and Mirski, 1998) (see Table 16.2.).

TABLE 16.2. Neurotransmitter Actions of Drugs Used to Curb Violence in Patients

	Dopamine	Serotonin	GABA	Norepi-nephrine	Acetylcho-line
Benzodiazepines			+++		
Antipsychotics	---	+			---
Trazodone		+++			---
Buspirone		+++			
Propranolol				---	
Valproic acid		+	+		
Carbamezapine			+		---

+ = Enhancement; - = Blockage

When evaluating open trials and also in clinical practice, it should be borne in mind that there is a tendency toward spontaneous improvement of conditions of violence. Nilsson, Palmstierna, and Wisted (1988) recommend a long "run-in" period with two or three weeks of observation before introducing any kind of active treatment.

Halivan

The combination of haloperidol and a short-acting benzodiazepine, often referred to as "Halivan," is probably the market leader for emergency sedation. Thacker (1996) presented the following case vignette to a group of British doctors and asked their opinions about psychopharmacological management:

A previously healthy eighty-year-old man of average build was admitted today with a chest infection, severe dehydration, and confusion. He requires fluids and antibiotics urgently, but offers of oral medication have been thwarted by threats and punches. All attempts to orientate and reassure him have failed.

The most popular drugs for initial use were intramuscular haloperidol alone in doses up to 5 mg, intramuscular or lorazepam alone in doses up to 4 mg. Yudovsky, Silver, and Hales (1990), based on their clinical experience, suggest initial use of haloperidol (Haldol) 1 mg by mouth or .5 mg intravenous or intramuscular, repeated every hour until control of aggression is achieved. If lorazepam (Ativan) is used, they suggest 1-2 mg by mouth or intramuscular repeated every hour until the patient is calm. A maximum dose of 5 mg of intramuscular haloperidol is recommended by the manufacturer for severely agitated patients, and a maximum dose of 4 mg for lorazepam. These are doses recommended when given separately and no intramuscular geriatric dosages are established.

Intravenous use of haloperidol does not have Food and Drug Administration approval, is seldom practical in the nursing home, and can cause cardiac arrhythmias (Sharma et al., 1998). Geriatric experience with droperidol, a related butyrophenone that has been used for combative patients (Thomas, Schwartz, and Petrilli, 1992), is limited.

Benzodiazepines are indicated in delirium caused by withdrawal of alcohol or of benzodiazepines but may, in fact, because of their disinhibiting effect, contribute to increased violence. In practice they are often used in the agitated elderly, sometimes with the rationale that the agitation is due to anxiety (Billig, Cohen-Mansfield, and Lipson, 1991).

Carbamezapine

The efficacy of carbamezapine (Tegretol) in mania, and in episodic violence associated with complex seizures, has led to consideration of its use in other forms of violence (Patterson, 1987). Its side effects include dizziness, ataxia, and production of blood, liver, and cardiac abnormalities. Marin and Greenwald (1989) have suggested that carbamezapine is of particular use for those who are resistive during care.

Trazodone

Trazodone (Desyrel) is one of several antidepressant drugs that inhibit the reuptake of serotonin. As compared with other serotonergic antidepressants, it has a sedating effect. This combination of properties has led to its consideration as a drug for aggression. Houlihan and colleagues (1994) reviewed the previous work on the use of the drug in dementia and carried out an open trial. They found that the drug produced general behavioral improvement in dementia, but had no specific effect on hostility. Improvement in this trial and in that of Pinner and Rich (1988) took several weeks. Greenwald, Marin, and Silverman (1986) described an eighty-two-year-old patient with repetitive screaming and table and head banging who responded over a six-week period to trazodone, accompanied by the serotonin precursor L-tryptophan.

Buspirone

Buspirone (Buspar) has been shown in animal studies to reduce aggression and to have serotonergic properties. Based on these observations, Herrmann and Eryavec (1993) used the drug with some success in sixteen psychogeriatric patients with agitation and depression that had not responded to previous treatment. Lawlor (1998) in a double-blind study, found that buspirone showed no advantage over placebo, and was inferior to trazodone in behaviorally disturbed Alzheimer patients.

Propranolol

Propranolol (Inderal) is a nonselective ß-blocker. Yudofsky, Williams, and Gorman (1981) described successful use of propranolol in four patients with outbursts of uncontrollable rage. They recommend an eight-week trial of its use in selected elderly patients, without cardiovascular or pulmonary disorder, with chronic aggression.

Valproic Acid

Valproic acid (Depakene) has antiepileptic and antimanic properties, probably related to an action on GABA (γ-aminobutyric acid) nerve cell receptors. It may also enhance serotonergic neurotransmission (McElroy et al., 1996). Divalproex sodium (Depakote) is a stable combination compound of valproic acid and sodium valproate. Its use to curb agitation in geriatric patients has been recommended on the basis of open trials (Porsteinsson et al., 1997). Gardner, Ditmanson, and Baker (1998), from a retrospective chart study of thirteen patients, suggest that it is useful in the treatment of aggressive behaviors in dementia. A summary of evidence for drug use in violence in specific concerns in the elderly is presented in Table 16.3.

TABLE 16.3. Evidence for Drugs Used in Violence and Specific Concerns in the Elderly

	Types of Evidence	Specific Concerns in the Elderly
Benzodiazepines	clinical experience, consensus	falls, cognitive impairment
Dopamine-blocking antipsychotics	clinical experience, consensus, controlled trials	falls, tardive dyskinesia, cognitive impairment
Trazodone	open trials	drowsiness may lead to falls
Buspirone	animal studies, open trial	
Propranolol	open trial	cardiovascular and respiratory effects
Valproic acid	open trials in agitated dementia, retrospective chart study in violent nursing home patients	
Carbamezapine	controlled trials in mania and complex seizures, anecdotal evidence in elderly	anticholinergic effects

Chapter 17

Nonviolent Antisocial Behaviors

Nursing home residents often show behavior disturbances that do not fall into any recognized psychiatric category or conform to any specific diagnosis. Apart from wandering and physical violence, patients who bother other patients, their families, and the staff may do so in a variety of ways. Among those noted by Zimmer, Watson, and Treat (1984) in a random sample of Upstate New York nursing homes were spitting out medication, throwing food or objects, unfastening others' restraints, dangerous smoking habits, removing catheters, taking others' belongings, urinating in wastepaper baskets, smearing feces, public masturbation, and hoarding. These authors comment that the small proportion of offenders makes disproportionate demands on staff. "In facilities which are accustomed to a clientele composed of physically disabled elderly patients without significant behavioral problems even one or two severely disturbed patients would provide a disproportionately great burden of care on staff" (p. 1119).

The question of what constitutes a disturbed behavior is not always simple. It is largely a matter of context. Nursing home staff are commonly not bothered too much by the mere presence of delusions or halucinations, although the family may get very upset. Requests for psychiatric consultation emanating from the nursing home staff usually relate to behavior that is antisocial or difficult to deal with, although this behavior can in turn be based on delusions or hallucinations.

The traditions of the nursing home derive from the acute care general hospital. Patients are expected to go to bed early (often inordinately early) and then stay there. When the focus is upon physical measures, such as the giving of medication and the taking of temperatures, patients who do not cooperate with the procedures are disruptive. As in the case described in Chapter 16, simple actions such as walking into the nursing station or lying on the floor can be a tremendously disruptive behavior in some medical contexts but cause no disturbance in others. Loss of capacity for ADL is commonly well-tolerated by nursing home staffing but disruptive to the life of family caregivers when the patient is at home.

For every disturbing behavior there is someone who is disturbed by it, and identifying who that disturbed person or persons is may be a first step in dealing with the behavior.

AGITATION

A symptom or behavior that is often mentioned in nursing home patients is "agitation." Strictly speaking, and having regard to etymology, it is used to describe states of increased motor activity accompanied by a negative mood, but it is not really a technical psychiatric term. It is used colloquially in various senses. A patient in my office recently said she felt agitated. When I asked her what she meant, she said, "I feel like I want to jump out of my skin." Many of us might describe ourselves as feeling "agitated" in certain circumstances even if we are not moving around. It would be, for us, an unpleasant state of mind in which we were unable to rest or concentrate.

The word is commonly used by staff in health care settings to describe demented and elderly patients, rather than the young and vioent. When used to describe behavior, it implies that the patient can talk or move about. The mute and immobile are not described as agitated, although they may feel inwardly agitated. Patients who wander, patients who shout, patients who cry, and patients who resist care may all be described as agitated. Agitation may, in fact, be used by nursing home staff as a portmanteau word to describe undesirable behavior. Because of this loose usage, attempts have been made to define and measure the components of agitation. Defining the problem exactly can be helpful in formulating treatment plans.

According to Cohen-Mansfield (1986) the definition of agitation is "inappropriate verbal, vocal, or motor activity that is not explained by needs or confusion per se. It includes behavior such as aimless wandering, pacing, cursing, screaming, biting, and fighting" (p. 722). From analysis of data from nursing home patients she was able to group agitated behaviors into four factors or syndromes of agitation:

aggressive-physical, aggressive-verbal, hoarding, and nonaggressive. The nonaggressive syndrome was characterized particularly by pacing, inappropriate dressing or disrobing, and requests for attention.

Other writers have found slightly different groupings of symptoms. Rohrer, Buckwalter, and Russell (1989) analyzed the behavior of 285 nursing home residents and found that the disturbed behaviors that affected the amount of care needed could be described in terms of three factors: cognitive defects, negative affect, and aggressiveness.

The Pittsburgh Agitation Scale (Rosen et al., 1994) measures four groups of agitated behaviors: aberrant vocalization, motor agitation, aggressiveness, and resisting care (see Table 17.1).

Sundowning

A separate entity of "senile nocturnal delirium" was described by Cameron in 1941, and many of those caring for the aged since have described a phenomenon they refer to as "sundowning" (Evans, 1987), in which agitation increases as night approaches.

Belief in this entity is stronger than the experimental evidence for its existence. Bliwise and colleagues (1993) suggest that "at least some components of sundowning may reflect disruptive behaviors that occur with identical frequency throughout the day but with differential impact on nursing staff" (p. 790). These investigators found that awakening from sleep in darkness associates with agitation in demented nursing home patients.

Does Psychiatric Diagnosis Matter?

Classifications of agitated behavior often ignore diagnoses. Dementia is probably the most common associated condition, but the presence and severity of agitation do not correlate well with the seerity of dementia. It is probable (although difficult to prove) that the presence of cognitive impairment operates to convert the symptomatology of several psychiatric and medical conditions to agitation. Thus, a condition such as anxiety or mania in a demented patient can appear as agitation.

Nonpsychiatric medical diagnoses can also enter into this pathoplastic disease/disease interaction. In delirium, the physical distress caused by the general medical condition is a factor in agitation.

TABLE 17.1. Pittsburgh Agitation Scale

Behavior Groups	Intensity During Rating Period
Aberrant Vocalization: (repetitive requests or complaints, nonverbal vocalizations, e.g., moaning, screaming)	0. Not present 1. Low volume, not disruptive in milieu, including crying 2. Louder than conversational, mildly disruptive, redirectable 3. Loud, disruptive, difficult to redirect 4. Extremely loud screaming or yelling, highly disruptive, unable to redirect
Motor Agitation: (pacing, wandering, moving in chair, taking others' possessions. Rate "intrusiveness" by normal social standards, not by effect on others in milieu. If "intrusive" or "disruptive" due to noise, rate under "vocalization")	0. Not present 1. Pacing or moving about in a chair at normal rate (appears to be seeking comfort, looking for spouse, purposeless movements) 2. Increased rate of movements, mildly intrusive, easily redirectable 3. Rapid movements, moderately intrusive or disruptive, difficult to redirect 4. Intense movements, extremely intrusive or disruptive, not redirectable verbally
Aggressiveness: (score "0" if aggressive only when resisting care)	0. Not present 1. Verbal threats 2. Threatening gestures; no attempt to strike 3. Physical toward property 4. Physical toward self or others
Resisting Care: Washing Dressing Eating Meds Other	0. Not present 1. Procrastination or avoidance 2. Verbal/gesture of refusal 3. Pushing away to avoid task 4. Striking out at caregiver

Source: Rosen et al., 1994, p. 58.

Alzheimer's Disease and Behavior Disturbance

Attempts to classify the behavior disturbances of Alzheimer's disease and to assign them prognostic significance have produced inconsistent and contradictory results. Nilsson, Palmstierna, and Wisted (1988) found that aggression often remits, but Hope and colleagues (1999) found that aggression and loss of appetite, once they appear characteristically, persist until death. Among demented outpatients studied by Swearer and colleagues (1988), angry outbursts were the most prevalent type of disturbed behavior. These were often accompanied by physical aggression and by anxiety, but showed no correlation with paranoid delusions or hallucinations. They increased with the severity of the dementia. Sleep disturbance and appetite disturbance tended to go together but were not correlated with severity of dementia. Harwood and colleagues (1998) found five clusters of behavioral symptoms among Alzheimer's patients attending a memory disorder clinic (see Table 17.2).

In this study the "psychosis" group of symptoms predicted a faster decline in cognitive functions.

Management of Agitation

The treatment of agitation needs a multidisciplinary approach with contributions from all disciplines. When the care plan is formulated agitation should be approached by breaking it down into its component behaviors and emotional states. The same principle may be applied to all kinds of disruptive behavior. Is the behavior really disruptive, and if so, to whom? Is the patient wandering or shouting? Is he or she weeping? Is he or she angry, frightened, fearful, or overly cheerful? Is

TABLE 17.2. Behavior Disorders in Alzheimer's Disease

Agitation/anxiety	Agitation
	Anxiety of upcoming events
	Other anxiety
Psychosis	Delusions of theft
	Suspiciousness/paranoia
	Visual hallucinations
Aggression	Verbal aggression
	Physical threats/violence
	Fear of being left alone
	Other delusions
Depression	Tearfulness
	Depressed mood
Activity disturbance	Wandering
	Delusion one's house is not one's home

Source: Harwood et al., 1998.

he or she hallucinating? For each obviously abnormal behavior it is then necessary to ask, in a tactful way, who is being upset by it. Often this question has not been previously considered, and looking for the answer is the solution. A list of those upset must be compiled, and each individual or group considered separately. With this analysis, a set of measures can be initiated to address particular problems.

Medication

A large number of drugs have been used to manage agitation. The evidence from controlled trials is scanty and suggests that the drugs largely act, if at all, as nonspecific sedatives, except in those cases indicating a specific definite psychiatric diagnosis. The drugs have included buspirone, lorazepam, olanzapine, risperidone, fluphenazine, and trazodone (Alexopoulos et al., 1998; Work Group on Alzheimer's Disease and Related Dementias, 1997).

Christensen and Benfield (1998) found no difference between low dose haloperidol and alprazolam in managing disruptive behavior in elderly nursing home patients. Claims for the efficacy of carbamezapine, valproic acid, and other anticonvulsants in the treatment of behavioral disturbance in the course of dementia have been conflicting and difficult to evaluate.

Herrmann (1998) treated sixteen demented patients with severe agitation and failure of response to other medications. Valproic acid (given as divalproex sodium, Depakote) was moderately effective over a period of four to six weeks (one markedly improved, three much improved, and four minimally improved). One patient dropped out because of diarrhea. The most common adverse effects were sedation and gait unsteadiness. Valproate blood levels did not predict response. Herrmann recommends starting at doses of 125 mg twice a day with gradual increase, monitoring for clinical side effects.

Goldberg (1999) used Depakote for twenty-two nursing home patients with dementia-related behavioral problems who had failed to respond to risperidone (Risperdal), and noted that twelve were improved. The average dose was 823 mg daily. The most common adverse effect was excessive sedation.

Probably there is a placebo effect on the caregivers. As with all drug use in the institutionalized elderly, a balance must be struck between those who are fearful of the patient being sedated and those who welcome a sedative effect.

DEMANDING AND DIFFICULT PATIENTS

Some patients are demanding and difficult to an extent that makes them difficult to manage, but do not have a specific psychiatric illness. That is to say they do not have an Axis I psychiatric diagnosis. The diagnosis of personality disorders (Axis II disorders) arouses even more disagreement among psychiatrists than most mental illnesses. Doubt exists as to whether Axis II disorders qualify as legitimate illnesses or are just labels for nasty or inconvenient people. Even more doubt exists as to whether they are treatable. Often this comes down to a "madness versus badness" kind of argument.

The present DSM classification divides personality disorders into three clusters. Cluster A are strange and eccentric but not quite schizophrenic. Cluster B are flamboyant and antisocial nuisances. Cluster C are not happy campers but do not quite qualify for any of the mood disorder diagnoses.

Disagreement becomes even greater when diagnosing the elderly (Molinari et al., 1998; Agronin and Maletta, 2000). Even mild cognitive impairment can damage judgment so that the impossible person is more obviously unreasonable. A memory impairment factor is especially evident in the common problem of the frequent telephoner. These telephone addicts call their families many times a day and insist every call is an emergency; they claim not to remember the previous call.

Some of these personalities have been difficult all their lives and their families became accustomed to them, but in the nursing home they have new caregivers to make demands upon. Their extra weapon is physical illness, which makes it more difficult for people to refuse them.

Nursing homes, in fact, are better able to manage them than are assisted living and board and care residences. In the nursing home the complaints are triaged by the nurse, who carries a certain amount of authority and can decide whether to bother the family or the doctor with a concern.

One of the assisted living residents rated as most difficult in an American Assocation of Retired Persons survey (Kane, Wilson, and Clemmer, 1993, p. 58) was described as follows:

Resident has COPD (chronic obstructive pulmonary disease); is demanding, harsh with family, staff, and other residents; alienating family; does not wish to get involved in activities; stays in her room; gets outsiders in an uproar regarding supposed health problems; doctor is continually kept advised of her condition; very unpleasant lady; can perform ADLs for self but tells daughter, "If they see that I can do it, they will expect me to do it all the time."

Managing such patients is often a matter of counseling others who must deal with them rather than prescribing direct treatment. In spite of the absence of an Axis I DSM diagnosis, the behavior can escalate and become so dangerous that hospitalization may need to be considered. For example, frequent telephoners may abuse 911 emergency lines.

NOISEMAKING

Noisiness and shouting is a common nuisance behavior in nursing homes, which has seldom been studied systematically. Sloane and colleagues (1999) found a division between "screamers" and "talkers." Ryan and colleagues (1988) divided noisemaking into six categories:

1. Purposeless and perseverative
2. Response to the environment
3. Directed toward eliciting a response from the environment
4. "Chatterbox" (these were the overtalkative; those who, once engaged in conversation, resisted attempts to disengage)
5. In the context of deafness
6. Other

They found about 30 percent were nuisance noisemakers. The most common category was "purposeless and perseverative," and this was also probably the most difficult for staff to live with, given the authors' definition of it as "behaviors such as moaning, screaming or banging which were persistent, occurred without nurses being able to identify causes, and in which noise-making patients did not respond to nursing attention" (p. 370).

Even without a loud noise volume, repetitions and perseverations can be difficult for caregivers to manage. In Parkinson's disease the voice is often monotonous, rather than loud, and repetitious demands may be repeated at an even pitch and low volume. It is often hard to say whether the unpopularity of some patients with Parkinson's disease is due to their neurological or their mental state (Gibb, 1989).

Causes

Noisemaking often occurs with dementia. It is especially common in the nonambulant stroke victim who combines dementia and aphasia. Ambulant patients with pure Alzheimer's are quieter. The more mobile the patients can be kept, the less noisy they are.

Banging and incoherent shouting can be manifestations of neglected communication problems.

> Psychiatric consultation was requested for an eighty-seven-year-old nursing home patient because of noisy behavior with shouting, banging, yelling, and what were described as "mood swings." She had been nearly deaf from childhood but had been able to drive and go shopping up until three years previously when her vision and hearing became worse. The behavior described in the nursing notes consisted of noise and screaming that might go on all night. She banged on things and clapped her hands and shouted that she was going to call the police and that her money was being stolen. She was able to control her bladder and bowels and feed herself. She was said to be unable to walk alone, but no diagnosis to account for this was recorded and the rehabilitation section of her chart was empty. The staff regarded her as demented, and had used several antipsychotics and benzodiazepines to treat her condition.
>
> On examination she was in night attire in a Geri-chair, and she banged loudly on the tray. I was able to get her to stand and walk, although she was somewhat unsteady. It was very difficult to establish communication because she was only able to hear a shouted voice close to her left ear. When I tried writing she told me that she could not see without her glasses. (The physical examination on her chart contained the annotation "EENT wnl.")
>
> She expressed resentment at having been put in the home, shouting repetitiously, "Who committed me in here?" She was fully oriented with no cognitive impairment.

Management

Environmental

Burgio and colleagues (1996) have pointed out the numerous methodological difficulties in attempting any sort of controlled trial of nonmedication interventions. The emotional impact of noisy patients upon the staff dealing with them every day can be great. This should be discussed in group sessions with the staff. Sometimes the visitors of other patients are upset, and they should be informed and reassured about what is happening. The impact on other residents is also of concern, but this is mitigated by the fact that so many are deaf or demented. Rooms can be changed around to make sure the noisemaker is not too close to any alert patients with good hearing.

Auditory Input

Nursing home staff usually try to deal first with the shouting by some kind of verbal method of discussion or reprimand (Werner, Hay, and Cohen-Mansfield, 1995) and it is true that shouting tends to decrease when the shouter is spoken to or involved in activities. A radio with headphones may be helpful. Burgio and colleagues (1996) used a cassette recorder playing a tape of ocean noises. However, this form of silencing is only effective at the beginning of the distraction. Therefore, a program must be worked out with the recreational therapist for frequent changes of the stimulus and of the environment. To take part in such a program, the patient should be alert and not oversedated.

Mobilization

Lyndon Johnson once described another politician as "too dumb to walk and chew gum" and many demented patients stop talking when they start walking. Even if a shouter is ambulant, it will often be observed that he stands still to begin shouting. Getting the patient outdoors is often helpful. This may be because the noise is diluted by the great outdoors or because of the distraction of the change in environment.

Medication

Medications are often used. These can sometimes help when delusions and hallucinations are related to the shouting, and if the medication is given in slowly graduated doses with the aim of treating psychotic symptoms rather than sedating the patient. Usually, medication does not do much good in repetitious shouters. Getting the patients so sedated that they fall asleep can produce all the adverse effects of heavy sedation, and the patient who is sedated to drowsiness on one shift may be back in full voice for the next shift.

DROOLING AND SMEARING

A variety of body secretions can add to the unpleasantness of caring for the institutionalized. The task of dealing with these is often delegated to the lowest ranking help. The patients are liable to be cleaned up by the time the doctor sees the patient so that he or she may fail to realize the severity of the problem.

Hawking and Spitting

Those who hawk and spit may often have physical problems and a search for this should be made. Demented patients with bronchitis or bronchiectasis may just get rid of their sputum on the floor.

A heavy smoker with a history of alcoholism and homelessness had been admitted to an inpatient psychiatric facility from an adult home because of frequent fights. The fights resulted from altercations with other adult home residents who remonstrated with him for spitting on the floor. The spitting was related to a productive cough due to bronchitis caused by smoking. He had a deprived childhood and led an isolated life without acculturation to norms of polite society. The bronchitis was treated, and he was kept in a nonsmoking environment. He was involved in group discussions on a therapeutic community model, in which the undesirability of the spitting behavior was conveyed to him. A goal of return to the lesser care level of the adult home was set in the psychiatric unit. Discussions were held with the adult home staff who agreed to his return if spitting had reduced to a lower frequency and if he attended an outside day activity. A specific length of time without spitting on the floor was agreed upon. Contacts were made to arrange a day program.

Drooling

Drooling can result from any cause of dysphagia, but the most likely in the nursing home setting is parkinsonism, and the most likely cause of the parkinsonism is the use of antipsychotic drugs. Even Clozaril (clozapine), which does not cause dystonia, can have this effect. Cessation of these drugs should be considered. Anticholinergic drugs such as Cogentin (benztropine) and Artane (trihexyphenidyl) are often useful but may, of course, have their own set of side effects and adverse effects (such as dry mouth, blurring of close vision, constipation, and urinary retention) and can potentially lead to delirium.

Feces

Smearing and handling of feces is seldom due to dementia alone. Its occurrence should arouse the suspicion of preexisting psychosis. One woman I deal with always signals her relapse into mania by carefully putting a film of feces over every surface in her room. She is not a popular patient but responds rapidly to lithium. The demented are seldom so systematic, but when mania is superimposed on dementia with incontinence of feces, the results can be quite spectacular. Another manic patient would prepare missiles out of handfuls of his feces and hurl these at staff who incurred his displeasure. The behavior disappeared completely and permanently when he was put on lithium.

Sometimes the combination of dementia, fecal incontinence, and immobility can cause smearing. Excessive laxative use combined with immobility can condemn the patient to incontinence of feces, which the patient finds frustrating, and thus reacts by some of the smearing activities.

A seventy-one-year-old patient was found "covered from head to toe" in liquid feces, while lying in bed. She had suffered a stroke with right hemiplegia, but remained able to walk with assistance, and had some useful speech. She was later noted to have fecal impaction. She then suffered a hip fracture and was operated on with successful union of the fracture, but she did not walk again.

Her medications included Haldol, 2 mg each morning and 5 mg each night; Dilantin, 300 mg daily; docusate (Colace), 100 mg tid; and senna (Senokot), 1 tablet daily.

Coprophagia

The eating of feces is sometimes suspected. It usually occurs when demented patients are lying in feces and put their hands into it, then rub it across their face. Frequent cleanup and avoidance of diapering will usually resolve the condition.

HOARDING AND RITUALS

Hoarding

Hoarding is common in dementia, regardless of cause, and often associates with repetitive behaviors, hyperphagia, and pilfering, although Cohen-Mansfield and colleagues (1989) found it was not associated with other antisocial behaviors. Delusions of being stolen from sometimes provide an apparent rationale, but Hwang et al. (1998) found that such delusions were not especially prevalent among hoarders. British and Swedish workers include it as a symptom of "frontotemporal dementia" (Lund and Manchester Groups, 1994).

Management

Hoarding is generally a mild antisocial behavior unless the hoarded objects smell or can rot. For this reason, nonperishables are often best left undisturbed lest they be replaced with more noxious objects. Providing adequate open storage space so that perishables are not secreted in dark corners is helpful. If enough staff is available, they can find where the things are hidden and clean them out at intervals. Such enforcement of tidiness must, as McCartney (1999) points out, have due regard to patient autonomy. Satiation techniques are sometimes useful. The hoarder is plied with inexpensive bulky objects of the type collected. There is little evidence of any benefit from medication.

Rituals

Ritualistic behaviors are often a simulacrum of previous work tasks that the patient can no longer carry out. Such behaviors may be innocuous but can be a nuisance. For example, washing clothes and other articles in the toilet, sometimes followed by attempts at flushing with resultant flooding, is a common behavior of the demented. Clumsy attempts at cleaning can include such activities as wiping urine off the floor with pieces of clothing.

Abnormal movements often occur in schizophrenia. They are stereotyped but elaborate and not completely repetitive. These days the distinction from tardive dyskinesia is often questioned, but the movements of tardive dyskinesia are simpler and usually limited to the lips and tongue. Other organic neurological causes include Huntington's chorea and hemiballismus following stroke.

Management

The skills of the recreational or occupational therapist are often useful. Fatis, Smasai, and Betts (1989) describe managing ritualistic laundering by providing a substitute activity of washing clothing in a sink. When the patient is psychotic and tardive dyskinesia is suspected, the only answer is to see what happens when the patient is completely off antipsychotic drugs for several months, but the experiment may not produce benefits worth its risks. Substituting an "atypical" antipsychotic drug for one of the older ones may be considered.

INCONTINENCE OF URINE AND FECES

Half of all nursing home residents suffer from incontinence (National Institutes of Health, 1988). The burden of incontinence on caregivers is so heavy that it is a major cause of institutionalization. Incontinence is a condition that transgresses specialty boundaries, and its causes may lie above the neck or below the waist or both. It is sometimes assumed that any case of incontinence of urine in an elderly persons with any mental symptoms is due to dementia, the dementia being of such severity that the victims do not care whether they wet themselves. This can ultimately happen, of course, and, since dementia is very common, cases of incontinence of urine purely due to the severity of dementia are not rare, but they are not the majority of cases.

In practice there is not usually one single cause of incontinence, but an interaction of mental illness and general medical and localized genitourinary problems.

Terms used in connection with incontinence include urge incontinence, stress incontinence, incontinence with overflow, functional incontinence, and neurogenic bladder.

Stress Incontinence

Stress incontinence arises in females as a result of trauma during childbirth and causes urine to leak with coughing or laughing. Some women have been martyrs to incontinence for years because of pelvic floor weakness, but have cleverly managed to cope with the condition and conceal it by a variety of compensating devices, such as frequently changing clothing and staying close to a bathroom. When a physical condition reduces their mobility, and a mental disorder reduces their faculty for concealment, then the effects of the pelvic floor condition become apparent.

Urge Incontinence

Urge incontinence is what the name suggests. It is associated with conditions, such as infections, that cause the victim to have to void urgently and frequently. It can also be a manifestation of the neurogenic bladder. Neurogenic bladder refers to the bladder changes found when control is lost at the spinal cord level. Some agitated demented women will constantly demand to be taken to urinate and will be found, on cystoscopy, to have low capacity bladders with trabeculated walls suggesting a neurogenic bladder, yet they respond better to behaviorally oriented treatment than to neurological treatment or medication (Lackner, Roach, and Kennedy, 2000).

Incontinence with Overflow

Incontinence with overflow can be neurogenic or result from obstruction to the outflow of urine. The bladder distends until it overcomes the obstruction and then there is a dribbling incontinence. Obstruction occurs in the male as a result of prostate enlargement or urethral disease. Anticholinergic drugs can be a factor. Obstruction usually causes acute distress in the male and leads to early treatment, but it can happen without articulate complaint of pain in the demented or drugged.

Functional Incontinence

Functional incontinence means that the function of the lower urinary tract is intact, but that immobility or dementia interfere with the ability to control the bladder. The victim cannot get to the bathroom or does not know how to get there. Incontinence in nursing homes is largely functional incontinence, as evidenced by the fact that it is strongly associated with dementia and the use of restraints (Morley, 1999).

Investigation of Incontinence

The investigation of incontinence in a nursing home has to begin with, rather than be supplemented by, an evaluation of mental status, and of whether there is awareness of loss of control. Medications must be reviewed. The mobility and ability to find and walk to the bathroom must be assessed. A rectal examination for an enlarged prostate is important in the male. The battery of routine admission tests will usually include blood urea nitrogen and urinalysis. Decisions about how much further to proceed with investigations usually need team discussion, unless the patient is fully capable of understanding and making independent decisions.

If any intrusive examination at all is justified, then catheterization for measurement of a postvoiding urine volume should be done. How far to proceed after this will depend on the particular case and the availability of urological consultation. A cystometrogram and cystoscopy would be the next steps along the line of full investigation, and usually means referral to a urologist.

Management of Incontinence

In practice, although investigations are recommended, it is seldom that specific treatment of a specific condition produces good results, except for the male with retention due to benign prostatic hypertrophy. Treatment of infections seldom cures incontinence. Most nursing home patients are not good candidates for specific treatment of stress incontinence. There is, in fact, a baffling tendency for the problem to get better with attention focused on it. This may be due to improvement of mobility, frequent escorting to the toilet, or ease of access to toilet facilities. Some nursing homes are more efficient in this respect than others. Some smell of urine and some do not.

Medication

Several drugs are used. When there is a residual urine then drugs that cause the bladder to contract more vigorously such as bethanechol (Urecholine) may be used. An opposite tack is to use drugs such as oxybutynin (Ditropan) and tolterodine (Detrol), which have a blocking effect by causing contraction of the urethral sphincter. These drugs have anticholinergic properties that can adversely affect cognitive function (Katz et al., 1998).

Prompted Voiding

The most effective part of most bladder training regimes is frequently taking the patient to the bathroom or "prompted voiding." This is helpful regardless of the cause of the urinary incontinence. Drawbacks are that it may be regarded as a violation of personal autonomy and can interfere with sleep (Cruise et al., 1998).

Diapers and Pads

If all else fails, then absorbent pads, garments, or diapers can be tried. These have many disadvantages besides their obvious aesthetic ones, but they should be available for patients who say they need them.

Catheterization

Urinary incontinence is sometimes given as a reason for inserting a Foley catheter. This seems illogical, since someone draining urine continuously into a bag can hardly be said to be continent of urine. Continuous catheterization may have to be used for obstruction when surgery is refused, although an ungrateful patient has often demonstrated the patency of his urethra by pulling out a Foley catheter complete with its inflated balloon.

The motives behind the widespread use of catheters are probably a matter of medical anthropology. Ribeiro and Smith (1985) found that one-tenth of patients in three nursing homes in Massachusetts had chronic indwelling catheters, with no valid reason in most cases. One-third of those who die with long-term catheters in place will be found at autopsy to have acute pyelonephritis (Warren, Muncie, and Hall-Craggs, 1988). They die in dry beds.

Incontinence of Feces

Incontinence of feces is less common and less well tolerated than incontinence of urine. If it is due to dementia, the dementia is very advanced and accompanied by immobility. Smith (1983) found that all patients with persistent incontinence of feces were "demented, very demanding, or both and were therefore unpopular with staff" (p. 695).

Incontinence of feces in nursing homes can be iatrogenic. Most nursing home patients receive laxatives. Some nursing homes have laxative orders preprinted on their order sheets or on rubber stamps, so as to ensure compliance with the laxative ritual. This ritual is older and stronger than medical science. It has roots in our earliest contacts with the controls imposed upon the developing child by the adult world. The belief that constipation is bad centers around ideas that toxic substances will be retained in the body if defecation is not frequent. Those who hold this belief strongly will, consciously or subconsciously, attribute many ailments to the retained poisons and will seek for themselves, or for their patients, a bowel movement every day. Querying the desirability of this can arouse strong emotions.

Many of the adverse consequences of constipation in nursing home patients result from the remedies, rather than the condition they set out to cure (Alessi and Henderson, 1988). Indeed, the only physical illness that can be laid at the door of infrequent bowel movement is often due to the prolonged use of laxatives. This is fecal impaction.

In fecal impaction, the rectum contains feces that are rock hard, called scybalous feces. Some such patients will also have the colon loaded with feces on an X-ray examination. (The normal rectum is empty on digital examination, and normally a plain X-ray of the abdomen will not show feces.) Fecal impaction is sometimes associated with a form of "diarrhea." What happens is that a very liquid stool leaks past the rocky feces. This can produce incontinence of feces. If no one bothers to do a rectal examination, and especially if the patient is too demented to complain, then the condition may be mistreated with antidiarrhea medications, such as diphenoxylate with atropine (Lomotil) or loperamide (Imodium).

SEX

It may seem puritanical to list sex under the heading of antisocial behaviors. Sex in the nursing home may have its positive aspects, and freedom of sexual activity is now regarded as a patient's right, but nursing home staff usually have conservative attitudes about sex, do not believe that the issue of sexual activity in a nursing home is important, and are skeptical about any attempts to change these attitudes (Steinke, 1997).

The most common sexual behaviors observed in nursing homes are handholding, touching, kissing, and petting. Most elderly nursing home residents do not masturbate or have sexual intercourse, although most men continue to have sex fantasies (Wasow and Loeb, 1979).

Sexual activity initiated by staff is rarely a problem. Touching and hugging are nowadays taboo in most psychotherapeutic settings, but some writers make an exception for the elderly and have actually recommended such procedures in dealing with nursing home patients. Possibly this is because they regard the demented as childlike, or they believe the elderly are so unattractive that no suspicion of impropriety can arise. However, even if this is so, not all residents are elderly, and there have examples of sexual assault and even impregnation of nursing home residents by staff.

A muscular, young African American was stricken by a stroke. After six weeks in a rehabilitation center, he made no progress and was relegated in despair to a nursing home. His left arm and leg remained flaccid and limp, but these disabilities did not extend to all his members. He aroused the ardor of an attractive female aide, who spent long sessions with him, to which the administration turned a blind eye. After a few months, by bracing his left side with the sheer muscle power of his right side, he walked out of the home to take up residence with her.

Behaviors that most commonly cause concern to staff are masturbation and sexual interactions between incompetent, demented patients. Many of the sexual misbehaviors of the elderly are non-orgasmic, without penile erection or ejaculation, and consist of touching, fondling, and accosting. This is frequent in institutions and female staff are likely victims.

Szasz (1983) identified three types of behavior among aged male nursing home residents: sexual talk, sexual acts, and implied sexual behavior. Some acts were acceptable and the upset caused by them could be reduced by staff discussion.

Management of Antisocial Sexual Behaviors

Management of disturbed sexual behavior should begin with finding out who is disturbed by it. Some staff are upset by the patients having any sex life at all. Tolerance may be considered but the feelings of victims should be carefully considered. Failing to heed the complaints of underpaid staff who need their jobs to survive can amount to harassment. Open discussion of attitudes among staff can increase comfort with sexual issues. A useful approach in meetings is to present a scenario or case history and encourage participants to share how they would intervene.

Behavior such as persistent open masturbation can be difficult for the most broad-minded to tolerate. Such disinhibited actions may be especially common with right frontal brain lesions, but in most cases specific neurological or endocrinological abnormality can be found.

Medication

Use of antiandrogenic medication remains controversial (Jensen, 1989) because such treatment can theoretically produce chemical castration and eliminate all sexual pleasure. On the other hand, it has been argued (Cooper, 1987) that the demented elderly are inundated with drugs anyway, and these are more harmless than most.

Levitsky and Owens (1999) have reviewed the pharmacologic treatment of hypersexuality and paraphilias in nursing home residents. No placebo-controlled double-blind trials in elderly males were reported. Antiandrogens (six cases), estrogens (forty cases), gonadotrophin-releasing hormone analogs (one case in a forty-three-year-old with dementia), and antidepressant drugs (three cases) have been used. Aberrant male sex behaviors in the elderly are often nonorgasmic; that is to say they do not culminate in erection and ejaculation. It might be expected that medications that prevent arousal would be more useful in orgasmic behaviors.

Stewart and Shin (1997) reported a sixty-nine-year-old demented patient living in an assisted living facility whose behaviors included fondling or exposing himself to female patients, staff, and visitors; masturbating in public; and repeated graphic requests for sexual favors. He had failed to respond to a variety of psychotropic drugs (haloperidol, thioridazine, lorazepam, lithium, and amitriptyline). One week after starting 20 mg per day of paroxetine (Paxil), these behaviors had improved "around 95 percent" in the estimation of staff, and the improvement had been maintained for three months at the time of reporting.

Raji, Liu, and Wallace (2000) described a ninety-year-old female nursing home patient with sexual aggression. She would disrobe and grab at men's pelvic areas and would kick and hit when her sexual advances were rejected. She failed to respond to valproic acid or paroxetine, but improved within a week after starting citalopram (Celexa), 20 mg daily.

Kyomen, Nobel, and Wei (1991) described a ninety-two-year-old widower in a nursing home with prostate cancer and progressive dementia who began to have violent episodes. "He forced his exposed penis into the face of a woman, and persistently thrashed his body against her. He approached other women, took their hands, and placed them on his body and penis" (p. 1111). Diethylstilbestrol was given and physically aggressive behavior reduced considerably after three weeks of treatment.

Chapter 18

The Medical Interface

MEDICALIZATION OF CARE

The reasons for placing people in nursing homes are many. These may include medical illness, but the amount of state-to-state variation alone makes it unlikely that this is truly the major reason. For example, in 1990, Wisconsin had ninety-four nursing home beds for every 1,000 people over sixty-five, but Hawaii had only nineteen (Marion Merrill Dow Managed Care Digest, 1991). Such statistics suggest that being in a nursing home is not a matter of objectively diagnosed physical illness. Differences exist in the distribution of disease, but not to this extent. Nevertheless, nursing homes are set up and staffed and financed so as to give a countertherapeutic emphasis to below-the-neck medical illness.

The interface between medical and psychiatric problems presents a paradox. Harm is done to the psychiatrically ill elderly by the medicalization of their care. Yet this harm is harm to their physical well-being. It results in increased death rates.

What are the modalities by which the process of medicalization harms the mentally ill elderly? Probably the poor results of nursing home treatments of the behaviorally disturbed result from a general feeling that all the elderly are senile and demented, that dementia cannot be treated, and that therefore only the medical aspects of their illness should be treated. This results in concentrating on the medical treatment of psychiatric patients while neglecting the psychiatric treatment of medical illness. Oversedation, use of restraints, and loss of mobility have been discussed. Polypharmacy is sometimes to be indicted.

Polypharmacy

One reason the effects of drugs may be deleterious among patients in nursing homes is that patients are more likely to take the drugs prescribed for them. In their own home, the elderly have the good sense to take only a proportion of the drugs their doctors think they are getting, although they are liable to counterbalance this by taking a few that their doctors do not know about (Spagnoli et al., 1989).

Oligopharmacy must not be irrationally elevated into a guiding principle. Careful care by conscientious doctors with geriatric expertise can sometimes legitimately necessitate the use of multiple medications (Rozzini et al., 1989), which are useful and necessary.

PAIN

Much of the psychology of pain is the psychology of failure to provide adequate pain relief. Nursing home patients often suffer pain, which is commonly left untreated, especially if they are black or very elderly (Bernabei et al., 1998; Engle, Fox-Hill, and Graney, 1998). This undertreatment is, paradoxically, probably another aspect of medicalization. The undertreatment of pain in the acute care general hospital was partly motivated by the sense of a life-saving mission. Pain might actually have diagnostic value. To get rid of it was mere symptomatic treatment unlikely to save the patient's life. Another factor in the medical hospital is the fear by doctors and nurses of being conned by addicts shopping for drugs. A fear more likely to affect the nursing home doctor is being accused of practicing euthanasia.

Some legal and administrative obstacles to pain relief are outside the control of the individual practitioner (American Medical Directors Association, 1999). In many states a nursing order for a controlled drug cannot be written just on the home's own order sheet but must be handwritten on the doctor's prescription blank. Another piece of bureaucratic idiocy is the "triplicate" prescription blanks profitably sold by state health departments which allow only a thirty-day supply of a narcotic.

In severely demented or noncommunicating patients, pain must be considered as a possible cause of behavior disturbance.

A nursing home patient began to have outbursts of disturbed behavior at mealtimes. She had no understandable speech and had to be fed by hand. An aide noticed that the outbursts occurred whenever she was given ice cream, previously a favorite food. This led to a diagnosis of trigeminal neuralgia, which responded promptly and completely to treatment.

BEDSORES

The prevalence of pressure sores in nursing homes averages about 11 percent, but varies among nursing homes (Morley, 1999). This variation may occur because some nursing homes have different populations of patients or because some homes are better managed than others. The longer the patient is in the nursing home, the more likely the occurrence of pressures sores, with about 20 percent developing one sore after two years (Bennett et al., 2000). The patient behavior associated with pressure sores is loss of mobility, especially becoming bedridden.

Much is subjective in bedsore management. Many doctors and nurses have favorite recipes and schedules for preventing and treating bedsores and many new devices and products have been introduced. Few have been subject to scientific investigation (Ferrell, 1998). Those who develop special recipes for mixtures to apply to the bedsore may get good results because of their enthusiasm.

The pressure sore can be explained in purely physiological terms. When the blood supply of tissue is cut off, it is deprived of oxygen and gangrene sets in. Pressure on an area can cut off blood supply. Muscle is rather more liable to damage this way than is skin or fat or connective tissue. Muscle is killed if its blood supply is cut off for two hours. If the pressure on any one part of the body is over 32 mm Hg for more than two hours, then the blood supply is cut off and a piece of tissue dies. There are two ways to prevent this. One involves distributing the body weight over the chair or mattress so perfectly that no part exerts a pressure higher than 32 mm Hg. This seldom works.

The second method is to move every part of the body more often than every two hours, which is more likely to work. In fact, if a patient becomes fully alert and ambulant, the biggest and worst bedsore that ever was will heal without any medical or surgical treatment.

Why do patients not become fully alert and ambulant? Causes can originate from disease below the neck but in general, the causes are psychological, social, and economic. It is rare to see a bedsore persist in a patient who is alert and fully oriented, not severely depressed, and not being sedated or restrained. In dealing with bedsores the importance of mobility must be emphasized, but this must be done in a tactful way without suggesting any failure on the part of the staff. Guilt and blame can easily arise in dealing with bedsores. Morale is higher when dealing with bedsores that originated outside the nursing home and these are more likely heal.

AIDS

AIDS has not yet made the impact on nursing homes that was expected when the epidemic began, although one American in a thousand is HIV positive. The HIV-positive state is more common in the board and care homes. These are usually inner-city residents whose risk factors have been drug use and promiscuity, rather than homosexuality. This population exhibits many of the psychosocial problems arising from their lifestyles. Board and care home residents with suspect illnesses often refuse HIV blood tests. The staff in the board and care homes are relatively phlegmatic about AIDS. This may reflect that they do not need to carry out nursing procedures that bring them into close patient contact. It may also reflect that they are so long reconciled to the idea of caring for those whom others have rejected, that an extra burden of stigma carries little meaning.

Why has such a prevalent disease not yet had a more severe impact on the nursing homes? Reluctance to accept patients may be a factor. Although overt discrimination is illegal, many nursing home administrators remain nervous about accepting AIDS patients. They may fear that staff will be lost if they begin to admit AIDS patients. Health care workers who have casual contact with, or provide routine care for, patients with HIV infections do not really risk infection (New York State Department of Health, 1988). Reassurances, however, are not always convincing, and one of the major psychiatric tasks in health care institutions is dealing with the fears of the staff.

Underrepresentation in the nursing homes may not occur entirely due to discrimination. Segregation may be self-imposed because AIDS patients are mostly young. The young who are not demented or psychotic do not want to be in the nursing homes with the old and demented. In some cases AIDS causes dementia. However, the life expectancy of those with AIDS dementia is limited, so there has not yet been a strong demand for nursing home care for this group. Otherwise AIDS victims, however depressed and demoralized, are cognitively intact and not psychotic.

Another reason is that AIDS care does not follow the model of care for the aged who are chronically ill. AIDS is an illness of long periods that are relatively asymptomatic, punctuated with acute severe illnesses necessitating hospitalization (Benjamin, 1988). As one director of nursing services put it, "AIDS is like a roller-coaster because residents can have a 103-degree fever, night sweats, and nausea for a day or two, then boom, they're going out to the theater the next day" (Mason, 1991, p. 37). Some are drug users. Some enter for short stays and are then released; they are often alienated from their families and need housing.

One answer has been for some nursing homes to specialize in care of AIDS, which can be an advantage in recruiting staff. Apart from fear of contagion, traditional nursing home staff experience stress from facing death and dying issues with this young population, and may be unsympathetic to their lifestyle. A cadre exists, however, of those who are well motivated to deal with these problems but would not relish coping with traditional elderly and chronically disabled nursing home populations.

NUTRITION

Obesity and Diabetes

Obesity is a particular threat in the nursing home because so many nursing home residents are victims of arterial disease, high cholesterol or triglycerides, or diabetes. None of them are likely to exercise vigorously.

Limiting food intake can be more difficult than ensuring adequate food intake. The obese maturity onset diabetics who eat themselves into hospital, and from there into a nursing home, have had a lifetime of practice in circumventing dietary restrictions. One obstacle is the sweet tooth that the elderly develop due to the atrophy of some specialized taste buds with age. The use of fructose and low calorie sweeteners may be especially useful for this (Endres, Poon, and Welch, 1989).

The nursing home offers an advantage over independent living or the general hospital when it comes to dietary treatment. Independent living allows unlimited access to snacking and hospital lengths of stay are too short for dietary treatment to have an impact.

Patient autonomy must be considered. Dietary restrictions affect one of the few remaining sources of pleasure. On the other hand, a low-calorie diet can be made pleasant and interesting. The patient's ability to make rational decisions must be assessed. Many patients will understand that the diet is prescribed for the benefit of their health. Those too demented to understand are not likely to overeat.

It is often relatives, and even sometimes staff, who question the need for dietary restriction and to monitor diet adherence. Our feelings about eating are affected by cultural background and childhood conditioning. Emaciation and failure to eat cause grave concern, but the risks of obesity are trivialized.

Pica

Changes in eating habits are common in dementia (Morris, Hope, and Fairburn, 1989). Sometimes the demented pull every object in sight to the lips and try to eat it. Many will eat with their hands. Pica, the eating of nonfood items, is commonly associated with very young children and the mentally retarded. When observed in the geriatric nursing home population, it will often be found that the patient has a history of schizophrenia. Nash, Broome, and Stone (1987) describe successful treatment by behavior modification of a seventy-year-old patient with this condition.

In practice, the knowledge most important in the management of this behavior problem is medical and surgical. Staff must be familiar with the danger, and frequent lack of danger, arising from swallowed articles, so that the patient is not rushed to the emergency room too frequently.

Weight Loss

The observation is often made that the demented eat ravenously while losing weight. Franklin and Karbeck (1989) suggested that the weight loss of Alzheimer's disease is due to a metabolic aberration inherent in the disease. The family is liable to say that the patient is not being fed properly, and the nursing staff and aides usually say that the patient is not eating well.

When patients fail to eat, the amount of anxiety aroused in the nursing home by food refusal is often disproportionate to any real danger of death from starvation (Norberg et al., 1988). Specific physical and psychiatric causes for weight loss should, of course, be looked for, especially depression.

High-calorie liquid foods with names such as Ensure or Sustacal are popular. They provide a nice aura of scientific medical treatment, although they are only logically necessary in cases of dysphagia where solid food cannot be taken. Favorite foods, ethnic foods, and foods brought in by the family can be tried. Wine is an appetite stimulant and calorie source backed by five thousand years of clinical experience. The dietician should form part of the treatment team that decides the care plan.

Tube Feedings

Arguments about tube feedings may be practical and may be philosophical and ethical. Ideally, we should settle the practical problem first before addressing the ethical question, but the two are not always distinct. We should decide whether the tube feeding will prolong life. This is not as easy as it sounds. Doubt exists about whether tube feeding is a lifesaving intervention in the demented elderly (Campbell-Taylor and Fisher, 1988; Gillick, 2000) but Cogen (1988) suggests that negative views about the life-prolonging efficacy of enteral feedings are motivated by a wish to avoid facing the difficult ethical issue. At any rate, both viewpoints should be aired during patient care plan meetings.

Traditional nasogastric tubes are only used on a temporary basis, for up to about two weeks. The classical gastrostomy involved the opening of the abdomen by a surgeon. The tube then passed into the stomach from the outside was usually a Foley catheter, which was held in the stomach by a dilated balloon on the inside end. Replacing the tube was relatively easy. When it was wished to try normal feeding, the tube could be removed and the opening would remain patent for up to several weeks if the tube needed to be reinserted.

It is now becoming more common to perform a "percutaneous" gastrostomy. A narrow tube is poked through the abdominal wall, into the stomach, without cutting open the abdomen. No major cutting or stitching is involved. These tubes have their advantages but they are not easily removed if they become blocked or are no longer needed. They are anchored inside by a latex plug, which takes a year to decompose. Usually the gastroenterologist has to be called when anything goes wrong with them.

Complications of gastrostomies include skin irritation, moniliasis, and granulation tissue at the stoma, leakage around the tube, and respiratory distress. The first action required when a gastrostomy patient is short of breath is to stop the feeding for a while, then recommence at a lower rate. If this needs to be done too often, the purpose for which the gastrostomy was performed may be defeated.

Gastrostomy patients usually die less than a year later, except in those cases in which the procedure is done as a temporary measure because of a recoverable swallowing difficulty, such as that following a stroke (Fisman et al., 1999). Death is likely to occur from a complication of the feeding tube itself (Thomas, Kamel, and Morley, 1998).

Chapter 19

Neurological Disorders

Any distinction between the spheres of psychiatry, neurology, and general medicine inevitably must be blurred and must often be arbitrary. The relationship between the two specialties over the years has rather resembled one of those Hollywood marriages in which the divorced remarry and then separate again. Illness is among the factors that cause people to enter nursing homes, and the illnesses most likely to cause institutionalization are those that damage the brain and affect the ability to cope independently with the complexities of life. Damage to the spinal cord alone can cause severe physical handicap, but this seldom leads to nursing home placement. Even quadriplegics can manage to stay home if they have enough money and family and social support.

COMMUNICATION IMPAIRMENT

Many nursing home patients do not talk. This presents special difficulties for mental health workers trained to use verbal skill, but such patients are not always regarded as difficult by the rest of the staff. The mute do not complain and are easy to ignore. However, they are in danger of losing their mobility and ADL capacity. It is important to have some systematic scheme for assessing the noncommunicating patient, particularly when serving as consultant, and seeing the patient only once. Ultimately, something intuitive is involved. The genius of Anne Sullivan lay, not in the particular methods she used to teach Helen Keller, but in her recognition that inside was an intelligent being. The problem, however, with pure intuition, and reliance on the glint in the patient's eye, is that it can lead us to confirm what we already believed. This systematic scheme need not adhere to any particular textbook, although it is often useful to say which tests were carried out, such as ability to repeat phrases, understand written commands, and name common objects. Any communication problem must be listed as a problem and addressed as a problem. Then it can be treated by the treatment team as a problem.

In the nursing home it is unlikely that a communication problem is due to one single cause. The causes that must be thought of include cultural and language barriers, dementia and other mental disorders, deafness, and aphasia.

Language and Culture

In an immigrant-based society, the elderly are those most likely to have retained the language of their country of origin but, for some of the reasons discussed in Chapter 9, the recent immigrant groups are underrepresented in the nursing home resident population. Communication barriers among staff and patients and families can arise when their ethnicity differs and may be attributed to language barriers but more often have their origin elsewhere—sometimes in racial prejudice.

Psychiatric Illness

The demented all eventually lose the power of speech. Those with Alzheimer brain changes retain the ability to read remarkably well while early on losing the ability to name common objects. Patients with alcohol-related brain damage show confabulation. That is to say they may be able to conduct interesting conversations about politics while being totally disoriented in space and time.

Schizophrenic and depressed patients who end up in nursing homes are usually the ones who do not talk. Noncommunicating psychotic patients may tend to get selectively institutionalized. They can present such overwhelming problems of medical, psychiatric, and social diagnosis that the only solution seems to be to institutionalize them, and then they, of course, make no vocal protest. Possibly prolonged institutionalization itself produces noncommunication.

Deafness

Even a relatively simple physical disability such as deafness has psychological ramifications. Obtaining a hearing aid for a nursing home resident requires an ENT consultant, an audiologist, and a hearing aid dealer, as well as determining who pays them. Hearing aid batteries must be changed once a week. The task is not easy, and a qualified staff member should be specially assigned to do this.

In a nursing home, many patients have $800 hearing aids that they do not use. They may or may not be confused, and it can be difficult to tell why they do not use the hearing aid. This situation can be frustrating, resulting in the staff giving up on attempts at communication. The potential for improvement by a hearing aid can sometimes be assessed by the old trick of putting the stethoscope earpieces in the patient's ears and talking loudly into the chest piece or by using an inexpensive hearing assistance device such as that described by Rizzolo and Snow (1989).

In theory, if the patient is totally deaf and wants to be cognizant of his or her surroundings, and can see and read, then a communication board should help. Ideally, this should be a large writing board with a big Magic Marker. It can be surprisingly difficult to organize this, and it will seldom be used. In fact, its main advantage will be diagnostic. It enables one to decide how motivated the patients really are to communicate (and how motivated the staff is to communicate with them).

Aphasia

Disease of the left side of the brain can produce in the right-handed a speech disturbance called aphasia. Inability to utter speech is called expressive (or Broca) aphasia; inability to understand speech is called receptive (or Wernicke) aphasia. More elaborate schemata, based on philosophical and neuroanatomical principles, have been devised from time to time to classify aphasia. It is important to differentiate aphasia from dementia. This is not so much because it leads to treatment of the aphasia itself, but because it suggests ways of communicating with the patient in spite of it.

Identification of the nondemented aphasic usually depends on some kind of test of visual memory. The services of a neuropsychologist or speech pathologist can be helpful in this differentiation but are not always available. Neuropsychologists are usually only available in teaching centers.

Speech Therapy

The role of the speech pathologist is largely diagnostic. The effectiveness of speech therapy as treatment can be difficult to demonstrate although it has been confirmed by recent meta-analysis (Robey, 1998). Once the speech pathologist has shown what the patient's problem is and has demonstrated how to communicate with the patient, the rest of the team must follow through.

STROKE

Disease of the arteries may cut off the blood supply to a part of the brain. The result may be to produce a stroke or dementia, or both. The dementia arising from brain artery disease has been variously termed "hardening of the arteries," "arteriosclerotic dementia," "multiinfarct dementia," and (most recently and officially) "vascular dementia." The word stroke is normally used for the physical events. In the most typical kind of stroke, a sudden loss of consciousness is followed by paralysis of the limbs of one side (hemiplegia). If the paralysis is of the right side of the body, then the power of speech is lost (aphasia).

Very often some recovery of the paralysis and aphasia occurs in the first few weeks after a stroke, but this period is usually spent in a hospital, and hope of further useful recovery has been given up when the patient enters a nursing home. Apart from dementia, a variety of psychiatric conditions can accompany stroke (Birkett, 1996). The emotional response may range from apathy to anger.

Depression

Depression can accompany strokes. The origins of this are controversial. Obviously, there may be demoralization due to the physical handicap produced by the stroke. The acute condition is often treated in the general hospital. Sometimes the patient is then transferred to a rehabilitation unit. The nursing home is usually viewed as the end of the line, and the patient who has retained good intellectual function may be painfully aware of this. Advocacy groups emphasize the importance of maintaining access to active treatment and rehabilitation facilities.

The depression may also have a more organic origin. Some writers claim that strokes affecting the left frontal areas of the brain are especially likely to cause depression, irrespective of the amount of physical handicap they cause. Those who favor this view tend to regard antidepressant medication as useful. Antidepressants, usually nontricyclic, are now the most common psychotropic drugs used in nursing homes, and are used most often in stroke patients (Lasser and Sunderland, 1998).

HEAD INJURY

Usually, head injury victims are young. When in nursing homes, these patients present some of the particular problems of the young patient in this context (see Chapter 9). The sudden transition to a helpless state is not only emotionally devastating for them but can affect the staff, who may need counseling and support. These youngsters are demoralized by their illness and by being in a nursing home, but they also suffer mental changes from the organic effects of their illness on the brain. Their behaviors are often delinquent and questions frequently arise as to whether these behaviors are direct effects of the brain injury or due to their situation.

Although their situation is particularly poignant, they also have more resources available than other patients, and caregivers should become informed about these resources. (<Headinjury.com> is a useful Web site, although run by a law firm.) The families and friends of these patients are more likely to be young and active and motivated to become involved in their treatment. These patients are not always dependent on Medicaid. Money may also be available from insurance and lawsuits, so that more intensive care can be given. Perhaps as a result of financial incentives, specialized units for long-term care of the brain-injured young have been established, and the possibility of transfer to one of these should be explored.

SEIZURES

Much has been written about the psychiatric aspects of epilepsy, and a number of psychiatric symptoms of an episodic nature have been attributed to seizure disorder. In the board and care homes some of these behavioral manifestations of complex partial seizures may be encountered. Also in board and care homes, alcohol use is commonly associated with seizures.

In the nursing home, the main epilepsy-related issue bearing on psychiatry is the use of medications. One-tenth of nursing home patients take antiepileptic medications (see Chapter 11). The most commonly prescribed are phenytoin (Dilantin), carbamezapine (Tegretol), clonazepam (Klonopin), and phenobarbital. Several of the older antiepileptic medications, and some of the newer ones, can affect memory and can cause drowsiness and gait unsteadiness. These effects can be increased when a psychotropic drug is added.

Age-related changes in metabolism and the use of multiple medications add to the complexity. The average antiepileptic drug recipient in a nursing home takes more than five medications (Lackner et al., 1998). In old age the metabolism of drugs is affected by declines in glomerular filtration rates, hepatic blood flow, serum albumen, and the ratio of muscle to fat (increase in the fat/lean ratio). The decline in serum albumen particularly affects drugs such as phenytoin and valproic acid (Depakene and Depakote) that bind to protein.

The patient who is admitted taking antiepileptic drugs may have been started on them for a psychiatric illness. Carbamezapine and valproic acid have now been in use for several years to treat bipolar disorders as well as epilepsy. Clorazepam and phenobarbital are used to treat anxiety. Newer drugs such as gabapentin (Neurontin) are also sometimes used for psychiatric indications.

PARKINSON'S DISEASE AND PARKINSONISM

Parkinsonism is a condition characterized by muscle stiffness and slow tremor. It is commonly produced by drugs, especially antipsychotic drugs that block dopamine. This is called drug-induced parkinsonism or EPS (extrapyramidal syndrome).

In idiopathic Parkinson's disease, dopamine is deficient in the brain because the part of the midbrain called the substantia nigra is damaged, and nerve cells contain Lewy bodies (particles containing a protein associated with cell death, called ubiquitin). Apart from full-blown Parkinson's disease and drug-induced parkinsonism (and a few rare diseases), many elderly people have slight degrees of stiffness and shaking.

Although the cause of parkinsonism is physical, the condition belongs almost as much to psychiatry as to neurology. Parkinson's disease is commonly accompanied by dementia and by depression. In addition to frank depression, Parkinson's disease victims are often querulous, demanding, and repetitious. Staff will often describe their voice as "whining." Further psychiatric involvement is necessary because the drugs used to treat Parkinson's disease often produce mental changes.

Lewy Body Disease

Lewy body disease overlaps with Parkinson's disease and drug induced parkinsonism. The victims suffer from dementia, which is often preceded by delusions and hallucinations. If given antipsychotic drugs, they are liable to develop EPS, even at a low dose. Their brains contain Lewy bodies.

Chapter 20

Death and Dying

One-fifth of us will die in a nursing home (Engle, Fox-Hill, and Graney, 1998; Fried, Pollack, et al., 1999). One-third of those admitted to nursing homes die within six months. Death and dying are, therefore, important topics in the nursing home.

Some therapeutic measures convey the image of being supporters of life very vividly. These are often the subject of laws commonly called DNR (do not resuscitate) laws. They comprise cardiopulmonary resuscitation (CPR) and ACLS (advanced cardiac life support). Such methods can, theoretically, recommence breathing and heartbeats that have stopped. They are usually all lumped together in legislation. In real life it is rare that a nursing home has CPR/ACLS capacity in the sense of being able to bring back to life someone with asystole or fatal arrhythmia. CPR in nursing homes is disruptive and upsetting for other residents, especially when, as is usually the case, it fails. It also wastefully consumes skilled nursing time, one of the most precious commodities in a nursing home (Finucane and Denman, 1989).

An informal element in DNR decisions in the nursing homes defies attempts at codification and formalization. The differences that can arise within a family can be beyond what legislation can provide for (Himber, 1989).

The ethical discussions may be more extended than insurance companies will pay for, and mental health professionals can find themselves involved in the rhetoric without being reimbursed for their time. Gillick, Berkman, and Cullen (1999) suggest that what is more important than specific DNR orders is having a general plan about intensity of care. They recommend allocating nursing homes to five pathways designated intensive, comprehensive, basic, palliative, and comfort only.

PATIENT SELF-DETERMINATION ACT

The Patient Self-Determination Act (PSDA, passed as part of OBRA 1990) was federal legislation meant to ensure that all people were given the right to decide what heroic measures could or could not be taken to prolong their lives. So many factors complicate the identification and interpretation of patient wishes that it is doubtful if the legislation is useful (Levenson and Feinsod, 1998). Teno (1998) has commented on the usefulness of the PDSA requirements with a quotation from H. L. Mencken, "For every human problem there is solution, which is simple, neat, and wrong" (p. 170).

PSDA required health care organizations, such as hospitals and nursing homes, to inform patients on admission of their rights under state laws to accept or refuse medical treatment and also to document any advance directives, such as living wills or health care proxies. Charts must be fattened in compliance with this, but no such discussions are really held with most nursing home patients (Bradley, Peiris, and Wetle, 1998), and even when they are capable of discussing it, many nursing home residents are unaware that they have a DNR order (Levin et al., 1999). Some of the language of PSDA is unclear in how it can be applied to nursing homes and is liable to conflict with state laws (Horowitz, 1992). So far, the assisted living and board and care homes have not been involved because they are not considered to be health care organizations.

DEMENTIA AND DNR

The interactions of dementia, death, DNR orders, and mental illness in the nursing home are intricate, and legislation has often resulted in further paperwork involving impossible psychiatric decisions. Most demented patients have sufficient understanding to appoint a health care proxy. This is a decision that actually only involves being able to recognize and name a concerned person who can be trusted to make decisions on the patient's behalf (Sansone et al., 1998). Ouslander, Tymchuk, and Rahbar (1989) examined how successful relatives and doctors were at predicting elderly nursing home patients wishes about high-tech medical interventions. They found that doctors tended to assume that the very old were less capable than they actually were of making their own decisions. Relatives did quite well in predicting what decision the elderly would make.

Sometimes the decision to withhold life-saving measures, or even an operation such as pinning a fractured hip, is made on the grounds that the patient is demented. When this presence of dementia is a consideration, then the doctors and nurses should be clear in their own minds that it is a consideration. They need not write down anywhere that treatment is being withheld because of dementia, but they should record the presence and degree of dementia. Dementia may impede active medical treatment in legitimate ways short of any kind of euthanasia. For example, the treatment may need patient cooperation, or the presence of dementia may alter the risk/benefits ratio. The life-shortening effect of dementia can reasonably be considered in making a decision about a treatment for a condition that would not kill the patient for several years.

In a nursing home where CPR\ACLS is realistically available, about one-third of patients chose DNR or have it chosen for them. Among those who have it chosen for them by a surrogate, very advanced age and the presence of dementia are the deciding factors (Fader et al. 1989).

Living Wills

In addition to DNR laws, "living wills" have been authorized by specific laws or by case law throughout the United States, Canada (Downe-Wamboldt, Butler, and Coughlan, 1998), and several other countries (Bowker, Stewart, Hayes, and Gill, 1998; Shields, 1995). Although the concept is widely approved of in principle, the number of people who actually make living wills is small (VandeCreek, Frankowski, and Johnson, 1995) and the impact on nursing homes has been slight. Those who make living wills are, paradoxically, more likely than the general population to die in a hospital and to be users of acute medical care. The high prevalence of dementia in nursing homes also reduces the number of living wills. Although dementia is not a legal obstacle to making such a will, patients who are cognitively impaired are unlikely to do so (Rodgman, 1996).

HOSPICE CARE

Most people prefer to die at home, but most of those who do not die in nursing homes die in hospitals (Pritchard et al., 1998). The hospice movement was designed to provide an alternative, although as yet few take advantage of it (Fried, Pollack, et al., 1999).

Hospice insurance benefits under Medicare demand that the prognosis is for less than six months of life, which is difficult to be sure of. Doctors and nurses tend to overpredict impending death (Finne-Soveri and Tilvis, 1998). Dementia is a life-shortening condition that may qualify for hospice care. In some studies, half of those diagnosed with dementia are dead three years later. The impact on length of life is less in the older age groups (Agüero-Torres, Fratiglioni, and Winblad, 1998).

HOSPITALIZATION OF NURSING HOME PATIENTS

The decision whether to hospitalize a nursing home patient is a more common dilemma than that of resuscitation. Every year 25 percent of nursing home residents are hospitalized (Gillick, Berkman, and Cullen, 1999).

Some families believe that putting their relative in a regular hospital is a guarantee that everything is being done. Sometimes the nursing staff do not have confidence in their ability to care for the severely ill. Nursing staff recently employed in general hospitals are liable to feel that it is neglectful not to hospitalize a severely ill person. In some cases, administrators fear that they may be held accountable for a death in their nursing home. The general perception of the elderly is that their illnesses are best treated in a hospital (Fried, Van Doorn, et al., 1999).

However, the hospital transfer is more likely to harm than cure (Gabow et al., 1985; Tresch, Simpson, and Burton, 1985; Sickbert, 1989). In acute care general hospitals, the confused are given tranquilizers; those liable to fall are put in restraints; those who do not choose to eat are tube fed; the incontinent are catheterized. These measures cause thrombophlebitis, pulmonary embolism, pressure sores, aspiration pneumonia, urinary tract infections, and bacteremia, each of which will, if diagnosed, be treated (Gillick, Serell, and Gillick, 1982).

Barry et al. (1988) studied elderly patients living at home who were so misguided as to refuse hospitalization recommended by their doctors, and compared them with a control group who were wise enough to accept. Six weeks later all of those who stayed home were still alive and still home. Of those who accepted hospitalization one-quarter were in nursing homes and one-fifth had died.

With few exceptions (such as the need for specific surgical procedures) the problem is psychosocial rather than purely medical. A variety of nonmedical considerations come into play and often cause conflict between administrators, doctors, nurses, and patients' families. (The patients themselves are less involved.) Families may oppose hospitalization because they are afraid their relative will lose his or her nursing home place. They may press unrealistically for it. HMOs have, theoretically, a financial incentive to avoid hospitalizing nursing home patients or sending them to emergency rooms, but this does not always work out in practice (Reuben et al., 1999). Medicare and Medicaid provide financial incentives to hospitalize nursing home patients (Ouslander, Weinberg, and Philips, 2000). The usual tendency is for doctors to want to hospitalize those patients whom the nurses believe should not be hospitalized (Wolff, Smolen, and Ferrara, 1985). This causes less tension than the reverse situation (Katz, 1989).

Dealing with these conflicts demands psychological skills. No one should be forced to experience situations they cannot deal with, but they should be given confidence that they can do as well as anyone else. It can be more cost-effective to set aside staff time to discuss these matters than to suppress discussion.

PART IV:
THE FUTURE

Chapter 21

What Is Wrong?

It is clear that something is amiss with the system, not only in terms of the care given, but because of vast and possibly unnecessary expense. One-fourth of those over eighty-five years old and one third of those over ninety are in nursing homes, costing $50,000 a year, mostly coming from Medicaid. The number of Americans in nursing homes is expected to rise from 1.6 million in 1990 to 5.3 million in 2030 and increase Medicaid costs to 75.4 billion in 2020 (Wagner, 2000). Questions arise. Must this go on forever? Is it an inescapable result of demographic changes?

What would be the consequences of the advent of an effective treatment for dementia—a magic memory pill? Several fantasists have envisioned utopias or (more commonly) dystopias in which humankind becomes immortal or gains eternal youth. It will be a long time before we have to cross that bridge, but a treatment for dementia is not completely beyond the bounds of immediate possibility. In the early 1950s, the idea of antipsychotic medication seemed remote, but within ten years of the discovery in France of chlorpromazine, the impact on mental hospitals was profound. Could an antidementia pill empty the nursing homes? If they were emptied, would we then produce the same problems as arose, or seem to have arisen, from the emptying of the mental hospitals? Must chronic disability always be with us? Has not the conquest of each illness—of tuberculosis, of syphilis, of rheumatic fever—always left us with new unconquered enemies?

RESEARCH

One answer to all of these questions is to say that we need more research. Nursing homes are tempting places for researchers, since they contain stable populations with difficult-to-treat diseases, skilled nursing staffs, and accessible records. The fact that most nursing home patients are mentally ill can raise ethical questions. In one research project, investigators from Sloan-Kettering injected live cancer cells into nursing home patients. When asked if they had told the patients they were injecting malignant cells, investigators replied, "Of course not; they would never have agreed to the study if we had told them that" (Cassel, 1985, p. 796). Such things would, of course, be impossible these days because of regulations such as "Common Rule," the Declaration of Helsinki, and the "Uniform Requirements for Manuscripts Submitted to Biomedical Journals" (Karlawish et al., 1999). Perhaps the pendulum has swung too far. If ethics committees are scrupulous enough, they can prevent almost any research. It is difficult to see how research on dementia can ever be done without using the demented as subjects.

Research on psychiatric illness is sometimes monitored more rigorously than other medical research because of an unwarranted assumption that mental illness necessarily renders patients incapable of giving valid consent to being research subjects. In fact, the research subjects in studies of medical conditions are just as likely to be incapable. In some such studies in which the patient's mental condition is described at all, such terms as "confused" are used without any definition or quantification. Less than one-third of the research papers about nursing homes in one survey contained any measure of patients' mental condition (Rabins et al., 1987).

The advent of the nursing homes caused a setback in psychogeriatric research in certain respects. Research in Alzheimer's disease is heavily dependent on autopsy material, and obtaining permission for autopsies on nursing home patients is difficult. The large state hospitals had their advantages for the researcher. The discoveries of Alzheimer, Simchowicz, Nissl, and other early German pioneers were made by doctors who were masters of both psychiatry and neuropathology. They had charge of their patients in large mental hospitals and followed their cases until the patients died, and then the doctors looked at the patients' brains at autopsy. Blessed, Tomlinson, Roth, Corsellis, and the other more recent British workers also had access to such populations.

Some methodological imperfections are intrinsic to the nursing home situation (Wayne et al., 1991). Control groups are complicated to arrange, especially for practices other than drug treatments. Much research centers around the areas of interest of academicians and drug companies rather than the areas of most concern to those who work in nursing homes. Some of the large tax-exempt nursing homes in metropolitan centers have formed strong teaching hospital affiliations, a development that may be useful for research. They provide teaching and research "material" for the teaching hospital (Libow, 1984).

There may be drawbacks to the academic orientation and some critics have been fearful of abuse by researchers, but on the whole, psychiatric research raises standards of practice and is helpful even if it does not lead to the discovery of the cure for Alzheimer's disease. As questions are asked about a patient as part of a pure research project, the answers will often suggest lines of treatment to the staff. The same patient who was avoided and regarded ás an untreatable nuisance becomes regarded as an interesting case to be studied.

Pressure for research in nursing homes can come from the families of demented patients themselves, who will want relatives enrolled in trials of treatment, especially new drugs. An ongoing research program offers a ray of hope to them.

THE VIEW FROM ABROAD

Is the development of the American nursing home peculiar to America, and is it due to the American health care system? Are the misplacements and overspending merely due to rivalries between state and federal funding agencies or are they an inevitable consequence of an aging population? Were mental patients dumped in the street by callous bureaucrats, or did these patients willfully fail to keep taking the pills that would have kept them cured? International comparisons are important in answering these questions. Certain problems are universal. Surveys of nursing home populations in Sweden, Denmark, Germany, and Singapore have shown underdiagnosis of mental illness, especially depression, in the institutionalized elderly, accompanied by overuse of sedative drugs (Hasle and Olsen, 1989; Lehmkuhl, Bosch, and Steinhart, 1986; Lau-Ting, Ting, and Phoon, 1987).

The British system is especially apposite because, while sharing a common language, the two countries have used radically different approaches to health care financing, and in Britain no dichotomy exists between state and federal funding.

Nevertheless, many of the difficulties in determining who cares for the demented elderly are replicated in Britain, even in the radically different administrative environment of the post-Thatcher National Health Service.

A specialty of geriatrics arose earlier in Britain than America, but it was a specialty concerned with rationing of care. With limited resources, Britain wished not to waste expensive acute care facilities on the old. Many of the hospitals that the National Health Service took over in 1945 were rather derelict places called city or municipal hospitals. These had once been poorhouses or workhouses. Typically, a middle-sized town contained the Royal Infirmary, which was more prestigious and did not take psychiatric or chronic cases, and the city hospital, which took all comers. With the advent of the National Health Service, these were supposed to have become equal but the public remained well aware of the distinction between them. The old city hospital contained so-called "part-three accommodation" in which dwelled the able-bodied indigent. It also contained the chronic sick wards, which were now designated as geriatric hospital beds. The doctors who had worked on the city payroll were now told they were consultant geriatricians in the National Health Service. Whenever new hospitals were built, or old ones abandoned (such as old tuberculosis or infectious disease hospitals) the older buildings would be designated as geriatric hospitals.

An alert seventy-year-old who fractured her hip and was operated on, would find that the next day, unless very influential politically, she had been transferred to the unattractive, if not insalubrious, surroundings of the "geriatric ward." Luxuries such as renal dialysis and heart surgery were not allowed for the old. A great deal of money was saved in this way. Britain is an economic model in health care. Health care in Britain uses less than half the proportion of the gross national product (GNP) than it does in America, and this is accomplished without any major differences in mortality.

Probably the long-stay chronic geriatric ward of the hospital was the most likely place in Britain to find the kind of patient who would be in an American nursing home. The patients in such accommodations in British hospitals were mostly demented and incontinent (Hodkinson et al., 1988). Many American city and county hospitals also contained such areas, and now sometimes designate them as nursing home beds.

Part III establishments were commonly called "old peoples' homes," or even, in deference to their historical origins, the "workhouse." This type of accommodation, run by local authorities, still has its counterparts in some county homes for the aged in the United States, but has largely been replaced by the board and care or adult home facility.

According to Perkins, King, and Hollyman (1989):

> Residential homes for the elderly are small establishments (usually housing 8-15 people) and usually consist of large old houses, staffed and converted in line with local authority registration requirements. Despite the relative uniformity of these registration requirements, such homes are very varied in standards, practices, and client group served. Some cater for more able elderly people, others take more confused and dementing residents. Often such establishments are run by nurses experienced in the care of the mentally ill. (p. 234)

While Britain does not have the American dichotomy between state and federal funding, the dichotomy between government funded health and social services has had a similar effect. The Department of Health and Social Services has been split into a Department of Health and a Department of Social Services. Health authorities have funding separate from that of social services departments. The Department of Social Services has a system of payments for residential care essentially similar to the way SSI pays for board and care homes in the United States. The mentally ill elderly who would previously have received mental hospital care have been thrust by health authorities into social service-funded homes. Fears have surfaced that death rates among those recently discharged from hospitals to nursing homes are unnecessarily high, and social services find their budgets insufficient to meet demand (Jolley, 1999).

There is, thus, a gradual rapprochement between the British and American systems. There are now many institutions in the United Kingdom that are called nursing homes. (The expression "nursing home" traditionally had a rather different meaning in Great Britain from America and indicated a small hospital, especially one privately run and outside the National Health Service, but the meaning is now changing more to the American usage.) These are privately owned, with many patients being paid for by the Department of Health and Social Services. This situation is very close to the situation in the United States where the proprietary nursing home contains Medicaid-funded patients. The British nursing home patients do not see doctors on a regular mandated basis and, in general, do not get as intense a level of medical care as those in the American homes (Hepple, Bowler, and Bowman, 1989). A recent innovation is nursing homes run by the National Health Service.

The overall picture is of less technology and less intense medical care. This began as a necessity, but eventually came to be seen as a virtue because home aides and general practitioners who make house calls are often more useful to the elderly than CAT scans and cardiologists. The British do use less psychotropic drugs, but this may be because they use less of everything (Nolan and O'Malley, 1989).

Probably the British example is evidence against the theory that the division between state and federal funding is to blame for the American problems. In Britain, as in America, the demented elderly fall in the crack created by the separation of social services and health care. The service received is often determined by chance, and by where the patients live or how they enter the system. It is difficult to distinguish among the residents of residential homes, nursing homes, and even hospital beds (Anderson, 1999). Acute nonpsychiatric care for the affluent young inevitably becomes separated from chronic psychiatric care for the elderly poor.

On the whole there is no one system in another country that is so perfect that America should adopt it lock, stock, and barrel as the answer to its nursing home problem. Mainly, international comparisons show how similar the problems are and how similar the snags are that arise in developing solutions to them.

Chapter 22

A Modest Proposal

The tasks of providing for the jailed, the handicapped, the homeless, the elderly, the addicted, the demented, and the psychotic seem inextricably and insolubly intertwined. The more services are provided, the more needs are uncovered and each of the needs is genuine. The more money is provided, the more money is needed. Measures to ensure that the money is properly spent involve spending more money. Many of those who help are overworked and underpaid. What should be done? Is there no solution?

IS HOME CARE THE ANSWER?

Home care is not the panacea it was once professed to be. When home care is at all intensive and professional it becomes more expensive than nursing home care. It involves paying doctors and nurses to drive cars.

One objection to providing nonprofessional additional home help is that it weakens the informal network of care (see Chapter 9). The informal network of care is an easily disrupted fragile ecology. If the state sends someone in to shovel snow off an elderly person's driveway, will the kid next door stop doing it? The answer to this question is elusive.

Home care is up against the economic problem of elastic demand. If home help is made cheaper, then people will want more of it. Many of the elderly would welcome additional help with doing their shopping or looking after their sick spouses if the government paid for it.

CALLING A SPADE A SPADE

A major error in current legislation is its attempt to get involved in psychiatric diagnosis. As we have seen, OBRA '87 reneged from its original aim of keeping the mentally ill out of the nursing homes. This was accomplished largely by setting up the dementia exception. There is no particular relationship between the diagnosis of the mental condition and the ability to manage it in a nursing home. Some of the demented are much more difficult to manage than some of the schizophrenic. The demented often, as we have seen, need active and skilled care for behavioral disturbances. Supplying such care would become easier without the Orwellian Newspeak involved in saying it is not needed. Improving government housing for the mentally ill may be an excellent idea. Changing the names for the housing from madhouse to asylum, to state hospital, to psychiatric center, and to nursing home may have been meant as kindness but creates semantic confusion.

MEDICAID SHOULD BE FOR THE POOR

The Medicaid-funded nursing home is the most expensive middle-class subsidy. The ethnic groups least likely to take advantage of it are those most likely to be stigmatized as welfare spongers. The nursing homes are sucking dry the Medicaid budgets. We should stop Medicaid funding for nursing homes, except for very severe physical illness. The states should be given mental health money to improve their state hospitals.

THE CHEAPEST GIFT IS MONEY

In general, the cheapest gift to give anyone is money. The demise of orphanages and workhouses may have owed something to enlightened benevolence, but was also because of finding that the straight handout, the transfer payment, was cheaper than providing institutional care. An objection to transfer payments such as government child allowances and tax credits is that they may encourage the improvident poor to beget more children. The supply of parents and grandparents, however, is limited.

I would give an approximate 10 percent increment in Social Security for every year of age after approximately seventy-five, and encourage the aged to shop for their own best bargains in nursing care and household help. Those who do not need any nursing care or household help could just keep the money. The reason for the age criterion is that separating those who need help from those who do not would involve an expensive bureaucracy. The exact percentage and age could be varied to keep this revenue-neutral. One objection to giving money directly to the aged and leaving them to do their own shopping in the care market is the belief that some of them are not sufficiently mentally competent to manage their own money, but many of the aged know the value of a dollar better than do the young.

ENVOI

Having suggested my own solution, let me conclude on a note of caution about all solutions. Let me draw attention again to the historical background described in my opening pages. History is the laboratory of social theorists and records many failed experiments.

Errors made in the past were often due to ignorance of the complexities of issues. Reformers would assume that problems were medical, political, financial, educational, social, moral, or racial and so forth. They would tackle one kind of problem and find that they had worsened another.

Many new initiatives to cope with the poor, the aged, the infirm, the mentally ill, and the delinquent have begun in idealism and ended in disillusion. Names that now sound grim, such as asylum, reformatory, penitentiary, orphanage, workhouse, and welfare, were once redolent of hope and kindness. "Nursing home" may be destined for the same linguistic ghetto.

References

Chapter 1

Federal Register (1989). Vol 54, No 21, February 2. Rules and Regulations.

Kidder SW (1999). Regulation of inappropriate psychopharmacologic medication use in U.S. nursing homes from 1954 to 1997: Part I. *Annals of Long-Term Care* 7: 20-26.

Medicaid Transmittal, May 11, 1977 A.T. 77-51, MSA Medical Assistance Manual: Mental Health Care in Skilled Nursing and Intermediate Care Facilities that Are Institutions for Mental Disease.

Smith EB (1998). Special report: Nursing homes. *USA Today*, October 13, 8A 9A.

Stotsky BA (1972). Social and clinical issues in geriatric psychiatry. *American Journal of Psychiatry* 129: 117-126.

Chapter 2

Beckwith B (1998). Washington Beat. *Geriatric Psychiatry News,* 9(5):3 November.

Borson S, Loebel JP, Ketchell M, Domoto S, and Hyde T (1997). Psychiatric assessments of nursing home residents under OBRA'87: Should PASARR be reformed? *American Journal of Geriatric Psychiatry* 5: 1173-1181.

Casten R, Lawton MP, Parmelee PA, and Kleban MH (1998). Psychometric characteristics of the minimum data set I: Confirmatory factor analysis. *Journal of the American Geriatrics Society* 46: 726-735.

Engle V (1998). Care of the living, care of the dying: Reconceptualizing nursing home care. *Journal of the American Geriatrics Society* 46: 1172-1174.

Finne-Soveri UH and Tilvis RS (1998). How accurate is the terminal prognosis in the minimum data set? *Journal of the American Geriatrics Society* 46: 1023-1024.

Kane RL (1998). Assuring quality in nursing home care. *Journal of the American Geriatrics Society* 46: 232-237.

Lawton MP, Casten R, Parmelee PA, and Kleban MH (1998). Psychometric characteristics of the minimum data set II: Validity. *Journal of the American Geriatrics Society* 46: 736-744.

Llorente MD, Olsen EJ, Leyva O, Silverman MA, Lewis JE, and Revero J (1998). Use of antipsychotic drugs in nursing homes: Current compliance with OBRA regulations. *Journal of the American Geriatrics Society* 46: 198-201.

Chapter 3

American Psychiatric Association (1998). Joint statement of the American Psychiatric Association and the American Association for Geriatric Psychiatry on the impact of the Omnibus Reconciliation Act of 1987 (OBRA'87) on psychiatric services in nursing homes. Presented to the Institute of Medicine Committee on Improving Quality of Life in Long-Term Care, March 12-13, Washington, DC.

Beardsley RS, Larson DB, Burns BJ, Thompson WT, and Kamerow DB (1989). Prescribing of psychotropics in elderly nursing home patients. *Journal of the American Geriatrics Society* 37: 327-330.

Carling PJ (1981). Nursing homes and chronic mental patients: A second opinion. *Schizophrenia Bulletin* 7: 488-498.

Citrome L (1998). The nursing home patient with schizophrenia. *Annals of Long-Term Care* 6: 347-351.

Goodman AB and Siegel S (1986). Elderly schizophrenic inpatients in the wake of deinstitutionalization. *American Journal of Psychiatry* 143: 204-207.

Harvey PD, Howanitz E, Parrella M, White L, Davidson M, Mohs RC, Hoblyn J, and Davis KL (1998). Symptoms, cognitive function and adaptive skills in geriatric patients with lifelong schizophrenia. *American Journal of Psychiatry* 155: 180-191.

Hollingshead AB and Redlich FC (1958). *Social class and mental illness.* New York: John Wiley and Sons.

Linn MW, Gurel L, Williford WO, Overall J, Gurland B, Laughlin P, and Barchiesi A (1985). Nursing home care as an alternative to psychiatric hospitalization. *Archives of General Psychiatry* 42: 544-551.

Loebel P and Rabitt T (1988). Nursing homes (letter). *Hospital and Community Psychiatry* 39: 997-998.

Redlich F and Kellert SR (1978). Trends in American mental health. *American Journal of Psychiatry* 135: 22-28.

Rovner BW, Kafonek S, Filipp L, Lucas MJ, and Folstein MF (1986). Prevalence of mental illness in a community nursing home. *American Journal of Psychiatry* 143: 1446-1449.

Schmidt L, Reinhardt AM, Kane RL, and Olsen DM (1977). The mentally ill in nursing homes, new back wards in the community. *Archives of General Psychiatry* 34: 687-691.

Shadish WR and Bootzin RR (1981). Nursing homes and chronic mental patients. *Schizophrenia Bulletin* 7: 488-498.

Snowden M, Piacitelli J, and Koepsell T (1998). Compliance with PASARR recommendations for Medicaid recipients in nursing homes. *Journal of the American Geriatrics Society* 46: 1132-1136.

Talbott JA (1988). Nursing homes are not the answer. *Hospital and Community Psychiatry* 39: 115.

Tariot PT, Podgorski CA, Blazina L, and Leibovici A (1993). Mental disorders in the nursing home. *American Journal of Psychiatry* 150: 1063-1069.

Teeter RB, Garetz FK, and Miller WR (1976). Psychiatric disturbances of aged patients in skilled nursing homes. *American Journal of Psychiatry* 133: 1430-1434.

Chapter 4

American Association of Retired Persons (1999). Assisted Living in the United States. <http://research.aarp.org/il/fs62r_assisted.html>.

Avorn J, Dreyer P, Connelly K, and Soumerai SB (1989). Use of psychoactive medication and the quality of care in rest homes. *New England Journal of Medicine* 320: 227-232.

Benjamin AE and Newcomer RJ (1986). Board and care housing: An analysis of state differences. *Research on Aging* 8: 388-406.

Bowland K (1989). Use of psychoactive medications in rest homes. *New England Journal of Medicine* 321: 54-55.

Braun JA (1998). Legal aspects of restraint use in nursing homes. *Untie the Elderly* 11(1),1-3 <www.ute.kendal.org>. Full citations from jabraun@ameritech.net.

Hawes C, Mor V, and Wildfire J et al. (1995). Executive summary. *Analysis of the Effects of Regulation on the Quality of Care in Board and Care Homes.* Rockville, MD: U.S. Department of Health and Human Services, Office of Disability, Aging, and Long-Term Care.

Kelly C and McCreadie RG (1999). Smoking habits, current symptoms, and premorbid characteristics of schizophrenic patients in Nithsdale, Scotland. *American Journal of Psychiatry* 156: 1751-1757.

Provider (1998). News report, December, no volume, page 11.

Pynoos J (1999). The future of housing and residential care for older persons. *Annals of Long-Term Care* 7: 144-148.

Rimer, Nancy (1999). A niche for the elderly and for the market. *The New York Times,* Special report, May 9.

Spore D, Mor V, Hiris J, Larrat EP, and Hawes C (1995). Psychotropic use among older residents of board and care facilities. *Journal of the American Geriatrics Society* 43: 1402-1409.

Stoecklin MT, Weaver K, Haan MN, Gilmer DF, Beck J, and Francis D (1998). Residential care settings in California. *Annals of Long-Term Care* 6: 342-346.

Vickery, Kathleen (1998). Medicaid: A growing payer for assisted living. *Provider* October: 12-13.

Chapter 5

Agronin ME (1998). The new frontier in geriatric psychiatry: Nursing homes and other long-term care settings. *Gerontologist* 38: 388-391.

American Health Care Association (nd). "PPS 1-2-3: What you need to know." To order call 1-800-321-0343.

Arling G, Zimmerman D, and Updike L (1989). Nursing home mix in Wisconsin findings and policy implications. *Medical Care* 27: 164-181.

Bartels SJ (1998). Funding reimbursement and public policy (abstract). *American Geriatric Society Symposia Highlights,* p. 16.

Beckwith, B (1998). Washington Beat. *Geriatric Psychiatry News* 9(5) November: 8.

Kane RL (1999). Future directions for managed care in nursing homes. *Annals of Long-Term Care* 7: 52-55.

Mirabile L (1993). The cruel cost of growing old just got better. *New York State Psychiatric Association Area II Bulletin* 35: 12-13.

The New York Times editorial, They didn't live so long for this. April 26, 1999.

Report by the Auditor General, State of California (1987). An Evaluation of the Medical Program's System for Establishing Rates for Nursing Homes. Office of the Auditor General, Sacramento.

Chapter 6

Loebel P and Rabitt T (1988). Nursing homes (letter). *Hospital and Community Psychiatry* 39: 997-998.

Long S (1987). *Death without dignity*. Austin, TX: Texas Monthly Press.

Mendelson MA (1975). *Tender loving greed*. New York: Vintage Books.

Mosca D (1999). Government is behind decline in care (letter). *The New York Times* May 2.

Provider (1991). News story. June issue, no volume, page 6.

Talbott JA (1988). Nursing homes are not the answer. *Hospital and Community Psychiatry* 39: 115.

Vinton L, Mazza N, and Kim Y-S (1998). Intervening in family-staff conflicts in nursing homes. *Clinical Gerontologist* 19: 45-68.

Vladeck, Bruce C (1980). *Unloving care*. New York: Basic Books.

Chapter 7

Bédard M, Chambers L, Molloy W, Lever JA, and Stones MJ (1999). The impact of Alzheimer's disease on caregivers is gender-specific. *Annals Royal of the College of Physicians and Surgeons of Canada* 32: 21-28.

Carnwath TCM and Johnson DAW (1987). Psychiatric morbidity among spouses of patients with stroke. *BMJ* 294: 409-411.

Eagles JM, Craig A, Rawlinson F, Restall DB, Beattie JAG, and Besson JAO (1987). The psychological well-being of supporters of the demented elderly. *British Journal of Psychiatry* 150: 293-298.

Molloy DW, Clarnett RM, Braun AE, Eisemann MR, and Sneiderman B (1991). Decision making in the incompetent elderly: The "daughter from California Syndrome." *Journal of the American Geriatrics Society* 39: 396-399.

Silliman RA, Fletcher RH, Earp JL, and Wagner EH (1986). Families of elderly stroke patients: Effects of home care. *Journal of the American Geriatrics Society* 34: 643-648.

Chapter 8

American Psychiatric Association (1998). Joint statement of the American Psychiatric Association and the American Association for Geriatric Psychiatry on the impact of the Omnibus Reconciliation Act of 1987 (OBRA'87) on psychiatric services in nursing homes. Presented to the Institute of Medicine Committee on Improving Quality of Life in Long-Term Care, March 12-13, Washington, DC.

Avorn J (1998). Depression in the elderly—falls and pitfalls (editorial). *New England Journal of Medicine* 339: 918-920.

Banerjee AK (1998). Caring for older people: 50 years of the British Geriatric Society. *Old Age Psychiatrist* Conference Supplement 2: 3-4.

Bartels SJ (1998). Funding reimbursement and public policy (abstract). *American Geriatric Society Symposia Highlights* 16.

Bartels SJ and Colenda CC (1998). Mental health services for Alzheimer's disease: Current trends in reimbursement and public policy and the future under managed care. *American Journal of Geriatric Psychiatry* 6 supplement: S85-S100.

Birkett DP (1980). The medical director in the nursing home. *Aged Care and Services Review* 2: 1-23.

Boult C (1999). Long-term care in its infancy (editorial). *Journal of the American Geriatrics Society* 47: 250-251.

Brannon D, Smyer MA, Cohn MD, Borchardt L, Landry JA, Jay GM, Garfein AJ, Malonbeach E, and Walls C (1988). A job diagnostic survey of nursing home caregivers. *Gerontologist* 2: 246-252.

Cadogan MP, Franzi C, Osterwell D, and Hill T (1999). Barriers to effective communication in skilled nursing facilities: Differences in perception between nurses and physicians. *Journal of the American Geriatrics Society* 47: 71-75.

Caudill M and Patrick M (1989). Nursing assistant turnover in nursing homes and need satisfaction. *Journal of Gerontological Nursing* 15: 24-30.

Cefalu CA (1998). Increasing the quality of medical care in the nursing home setting (letter). *Journal of the American Geriatrics Society* 46: 1327.

Cohen-Mansfield J (1989). Sources of satisfaction and stress in nursing home caregivers. *Journal of Advanced Nursing* 14: 383-388.

Deckard DJ, Hicks LL, and Rowntree BH (1986). Long-term care nursing: How satisfying is it? *Nursing Economics* 4: 194-200.

DeRuvo-Keegan L (1992). Letter from the publisher. *Provider* May: 8.

Elon R (1993). The nursing home medical director's role in transition. *Journal of the American Geriatrics Society* 41: 131-135.

Flint MM (1982). A consumers guide to nursing home care in New York City. FRIA, 440 East 26th Street, New York.

Gold MF (1999). A kindly touch, a helping hand. *Provider*. January: 56-59.

Goldman EB and Woog P (1975). Mental health in nursing homes training project. *Gerontologist* 15: 119-124.

Gurland B, Copeland J, Kuriansky, Kelleher M, Sharpe L, and Dean LL (1983). *The mind and mood of aging*, Binghamton, NY: The Haworth Press.

McCarthy JF, Banaszak-Hall JC, and Fries BE (1999). Medical director involvement in nursing homes 1991-1996. *Annals of Long-Term Care* 7: 35-43.

Moses J (1982). New role for hands-on caregivers: Part-time mental health technicians. *Journal of American Health Care Association* 8: 19-22.

NDTI Specialty Profile, psychiatry (1998). Plymouth Meeting, PA: IHS Health.

Reichman WE, Coyne AC, Borson S, Negrón AE, Rovner BW, Pelchat RJ, Sakauye KM, Katz P, Cantillon M, and Hamer RM (1998). Psychiatric consultation in the nursing home. *American Journal of Geriatric Psychiatry* 6: 320-327.

Saul S (1974). Group therapy in a proprietary nursing home. *Gerontologist* 14: 446-450.

Susman J, Zervanos NJ, and Byerly B (1989). Continuity of care and outcome in nursing home patients transferred to a community hospital. *Family Medicine* 21: 118-121.

Tellis-Nayak V and Tellis-Nayak M (1989). Quality of care and the burden of two cultures. *Gerontologist* 29: 307-313.

Tourigny-Rivard MF and Drury M (1987). The effects of monthly psychiatric consultation in a nursing home. *Gerontologist* 1987: 27: 36.

Turnbull JM (1989). The nursing home physician's image. *Geriatrics* 44: 83-90.

Watson R (1991). Meeting the challenge of a changing work force. *Provider* 17: 15-21.

Waxman HM, Carner EA, and Berkenstock G (1984). Job turnover and job satisfaction among nursing home aides 1984. *Gerontologist* 24: 503-509.

Chapter 9

Aging Health Policy Center, University of California (1986). *Improving the quality of care in nursing homes.* Institute of Medicine.

Bédard M, Chambers L, Molloy W, Lever JA, and Stones MJ (1999). The impact of Alzheimer's disease of caregivers is gender-specific. *Annals Royal of the College of Physicians and Surgeons of Canada* 32: 21-28.

Berthold H, Landahl S, and Svanborg A (1988). Home care and intermittent care. *Comprehensive Gerontology* 2: 24-30.

Breuer B, Wallenstein S, Feinberg C, Camargo M-J F, and Libow LS (1998). Assessing life expectancies of older nursing home residents. 46: 954-962..

Chiodo LK, Kantan DN, Gerety MB, Mulrow CD, and Cornell JE (1994). Functional status of Mexican-American nursing home residents. *Journal of the American Geriatrics Society* 42: 293-296.

Cohen CI, Hyland J, and Magai C (1998). Depression among African-American patients with dementia. *American Journal of Geriatric Psychiatry* 6: 162-175.

Crook T, Ferris S, and Bartus R (Eds.) (1983). *Assessment in geriatric psychopharmacology.* New Canaan, CT: Mark Powley Associates.

Folstein MF, Folstein SE, and McHugh PR (1975). "Mini-mental state" a practical method of grading the mental state of patients for the clinician. *Journal of Psychiatric Research* 12: 189-198.

Lathrop L, Corcoran S, and Ryden M (1989). Description and analysis of preadmission screening. *Public Health Nursing* 6:23-27.

Leipzig RM (1998). That was the year that was: An evidence-based clinical geriatrics update. *Journal of the American Geriatrics Society* 46: 1040-1049.

Lyons KL and Zarit SH (1999). Formal and informal support. *International Journal of Geriatric Psychiatry* 14: 183-196.

Miles F and Tisdall NP (1999). Reviewing admission policies under PPS. *Provider* 25: 4-16.

Retsinas J (1989). Helping families make the nursing home decision. *Geriatric Medicine Today* 8: 15-24.

U.S. Bureau of the Census (1993). *Sixty-Five Plus in America.* Washington, DC.

Weissert WB and Cready CM (1988). Determinants of hospital to nursing home placement delays. *Health Service Research* 23: 619-647.

Chapter 10

Arenson C and Wender RC (1999). Newer psychotropics and the older patient. *Patient Care* 33: 151-163.

Barnes R, Veith R, Okimoto J, Raskind M, and Gumbrecht G (1982). Efficacy of antipsychotic medications in behaviorally disturbed dementia patients. *American Journal of Psychiatry* 139: 1170-1174.

Beers M, Avorn J, Soumerai B, (1988). Psychoactive medication use in intermediate care facility residents. *JAMA* 260: 3016-3020.

Buck JA (1988). Psychotropic drug practice in nursing homes. *Journal of the American Geriatrics Society* 36: 409-418.

Burns BJ and Kamerow DB (1988). Psychotropic drug prescriptions for nursing home residents. *Journal of Family Practice* 26: 155-160.

Bushey M, Rathey U, and Bowers MB (1983). Lithium treatment in a very elderly nursing home population. *Comprehensive Psychiatry* 24: 392-396.

Colón-Emeric C and White H (1999). Case report: Catatonia and neuroleptic malignant syndrome in the nursing home. *Annals of Long-Term Care* 7: 28-30.

Federal Register (1989). Vol 83, No 25, February 2. Antipsychotic Drugs.

Glasscote RM, Beigel A, Butterfield A, et al (1976). Old Folks at Homes. A Field Study of Nursing and Board and Care Homes. Joint Information Service of the American Psychiatric Association and the Association for Mental Health, Washington, DC.

Helms PM (1985). Efficacy of antipsychotics in the treatment of the behavioral complications of dementia. *Journal of the American Geriatrics Society* 33: 206-209.

Jeste DV, Rockwell E, Harris MJ, Lohr JB, and Lacro J (1999). Conventional vs. newer antipsychotics in elderly patients. *American Journal of Geriatric Psychiatry* 7: 70-76.

Lasser RA and Sunderland T (1998). Newer psychotropic medication use in nursing home residents. *Journal of the American Geriatrics Society* 46: 202-207.

Llorente MD, Olsen EJ, Leyva O, Silverman MA, Lewis JE, and Rivero J (1998). Use of antipsychotic drugs in nursing homes: Current compliance with OBRA regulations. *Journal of the American Geriatrics Society* 46: 198-201.

Morgan K, Gilleard CJ, and Reive A (1982). Hypnotic usage in residential homes for the elderly: A prevalence and longtitudinal analysis. *Age and Ageing* 2: 229-234.

Peck A (1989). Nursing homes (letter) *The New York Times,* April 5.

Prien RF (1980). Problems and practices in geriatric psychopharmacology. *Psychosomatics* 21: 213-223.

Puroshottam BT, Keth GM, Gideon P, Fought RL, and Ray WA (1994). Effects of antipsychotic withdrawal in elderly nursing home residents. *Journal of the American Geriatrics Society* 42: 280-286.

Ray WA, Federspiel CF, and Schaffner W (1980). A study of antipsychotic drug use in nursing homes: Epidemiological evidence suggesting misuse. *American Journal of Public Health* 70: 485-491.

Ried LD, Johnson RE, and Gettman DA (1998). Benzodiazepine exposure and functional status in older people. *Journal of the American Geriatrics Society* 46: 71-76.

Waxman HM, Klein M, and Carner EA (1985). Drug misuse in nursing homes. *Hospital and Community Psychiatry* 36: 886-887.

Chapter 11

Ahmed Z, Fraser W, Kerr MP, Kiernan C, Emerson E, Robertson J, Felce D, Allen D, Baxter H, and Thomas J (2000). Reducing antipsychotic medication in people with a learning disability. *British Journal of Psychiatry* 176: 42-46.

Alvarez N (1989). Discontinuance of antiepileptic drugs in patients with developmental disability and a diagnosis of epilepsy. *American Journal of Mental Retardation* 93: 593-599.

American Psychiatric Association (1969). *Reality orientation. A technique to rehabilitate elderly and brain damaged patients with a moderate to severe degree of disorientation.* APA Hospital and Community Psychiatric Service, Washington, DC.

Beck CK (1998). Psychosocial and behavioral interventions for Alzheimer's disease patients and their families. *American Journal of Geriatric Psychiatry* 6 supplement: S41-S48.

Benson DM, Cameron D, Humbach E, Servino L, and Gambert SR (1987). Establishment of a dementia unit within the nursing home. *Journal of the American Geriatrics Society* 35: 319-323.

Berger EY (1985). The institutionalization of patients with Alzheimer's disease. *Danish Medical Bulletin* 32: 71-76.

Bettin KE, Maletta GJ, Dysken MW, Jilk KM, Welson DT, Kuskowski M, and Mach JR (1998). Measuring delirium severity in older patients without dementia. *American Journal of Geriatric Psychiatry* 6: 296-307.

Butler RN (1998). Brain preservation. *Geriatrics* 53: 3-4.

Cohen D, Kennedy G, and Eisdorfer C (1984). Phases of change in the patient with Alzheimer's dementia. *Journal of the American Geriatrics Society* 32: 11-15.

Crane L, Zonana H, and Wizner S (1977). Implications of the Donaldson decision. *Hospital and Community Psychiatry* 28: 827-833.

Denney NW (1988). A reanalysis of the influence of a friendly visitor program. *American Journal of Community Psychology* 16: 409-433.

Flacken JM, Cummings V, Mach JR, Bettin K, Kiely DK, and Wei J (1998). The association of serum anticholinergic activity with delirium in elderly medical patients. *American Journal of Geriatric Psychiatry* 6: 31-41.

Grant LA and Sommers AR (1998). Adapting living environments for persons with Alzheimer's disease. *Geriatrics* 53 supplement: S61-S65.

Hendrie HC (1998). Epidemiology of dementia and Alzheimer's disease. *American Journal of Geriatric Psychiatry* 6 supplement: S3-S18.

Hoffman A, Rocca WA, Brayne C et al (1991). The prevalence of dementia in Europe. *International Journal of Epidemiology* 20: 736-748.

Holden UP and Woods RT (1988). *Reality orientation: Psychological approaches to the confused elderly,* Second edition. Edinburgh: Churchill Livingstone.

Howell MC (1986). Old age in the retarded—a new program. *Journal of the American Geriatrics Society* 34: 71-72.

Lackner TE, Cloyd JC, Thomas LW, and Leppik I (1998). Antiepileptic drug use in nursing home residents. *Epilepsia* 39: 1083-1987.

Lakin KC, Hill BK, White CC, Wright EA, and Bruininks RH (1989). Longitudinal patters in ICF-MR utilization 1977-1986. *Mental Retardation* 27:149-158.

Leff B and Harper GM (1998). Case report: Exercising autonomy in an inescapable community. *Annals of Long-Term Care* 6: 439-441.

Levenson SA (1989). Synopsis of the federal regulations. *American Medical Directors Association,* Washington DC.

Lipowski ZJ (1983). Transient cognitive disorders in the elderly. *American Journal of Psychiatry* 140: 1426-1437.

Lund and Manchester Groups, no authors listed (1994). Clinical and neuropathological criteria for frontotemporal dementia. *Journal of Neurology and Neurosurgery Psychiatry* 57: 416-418.

Mace NL and Gwyther LP (1989). Selecting a nursing home with a dedicated dementia unit. Chicago: Alzheimer's Disease and Related Disorders Association.

Molloy DW (1987). Memory loss confusion and disoriention in an elderly woman taking meclizine. *Journal of the American Geriatrics Society* 35: 354-356.

Ohta RJ and Ohta BM (1988). Special units for Alzheimer's disease patienta: A critical look. *Gerontologist* 28: 803-808.

Poindexter AR (1989). Psychotropic drug patterns in a large ICF/MR facility: A ten-year experience. *American Journal of Mental Retardation* 93: 624-626.

Redjali SM and Radick JR (1988). ICF/general: An alternative for older ICF/MR residents with geriatric care needs. *Mental Retardation* 26: 209-212.

Riesberg B, Ferris SH, De Leon MJ, and Crook T (1982). The global deterioration scale for assessment of primary degenerative dementia. *American Journal of Psychiatry* 139: 1136-1139.

Sabin TD, Vitug AJ, and Mark VJ (1982). Are nursing home diagnosis and treatment adequate? *JAMA* 248: 321-322.

Seifert R, Jamieson J, and Gardner R (1983). Use of anticholinergics in the nursing home: An empirical study and review. *Drug Intelligence and Clinical Pharmacy* 17: 470-473.

Selzer GB, Finaly E, and Howell M (1988). Functional characteristics of elderly persons with mental retardation in community settings and nursing homes. *Mental Retardation* 26: 213-217.

Serby M, Chou JC, and Franssen EH (1987). Dementia in an American-Chinese nursing home population. *American Journal of Psychiatry* 144:811-822.

Stevens GL and Baldwin GA (1988). Optimizing mental health in the nursing home setting. *Journal of Psychosocial Nursing and Mental Health Services* 26: 7-31.

Utah State Auditor (1998). Review of the costs and services for individuals with developmental disabilities. Office of the Legislative Auditor General, PO Box 140151, Salt Lake City .

Wiener AS and Reingold J (1989). Special care units for dementia. *Journal of Long Term Care Administration* 17:14-18.

Chapter 12

Almeida OP (1998). Early vs. late-onset schizophrenia: Is it time to define the difference? (letter). *American Journal of Geriatric Psychiatry* 6: 345-346.

Carstensen I and Fremouw WJ (1981). The demonstration of a behavioral intervention for late life paranoia. *Gerontologist* 21: 329-333.

Harvey PD, Howanitz E, Parella M, White L, Davidson M, Mohs RC, Hoblyn J, and Davis KL (1998). Symptoms, cognitive function and adaptive skills in geriatric patients with lifelong schizophrenia. *American Journal of Psychiatry* 155: 1080-1086.

Holden NL (1987). Late paraphrenia or the paraphrenias? A descriptive study with a 10-year follow-up. *British Jounal of Psychiatry* 150: 635-639.

Jeste D, Palmer BW, and Harris MJ (1998). Response to Almeida. *American Journal of Geriatric Psychiatry* 6: 346-347.

Kelly C and McCreadle RG (1999). Smoking habits, current symptoms, and premorbid characteristics of schizophrenic patients in Nithsdale, Scotland. *American Journal of Psychiatry* 146: 1751-1757.

Mikkilineni SS, Garbien M, and Rudberg MA (1998). Case report: Phantom boarder syndrome. *Annals of Long-Term Care* 6: 401-407.

Pearlson GD, Kreger L, Rabins PV, Chase GA, Cohen B, Wirth JB, Schlaepfer TB, and Tune L (1989). A chart review study of late-onset and early-onset schizophrenia. *American Journal of Psychiatry* 146: 1568-1574.

Roth M and Kay DWK (1998). Late paraphrenia: A variant of schizophrenia manifest in late life or an organic clinical syndrome? *International Journal of Geriatric Psychiatry* 13: 775-784.

Rowan EL (1984). Phantom boarders as a symptom of late paraphrenia. *American Journal of Psychiatry* 141: 580-581.

Zinkin J (1950, translated). *Dementia Praecox or the Group of Schizophrenias* by Eugen Bleuler. New York: International Universities Press.

Chapter 13

Abrams RC, Young CR, Holt JH, and Alexopoulos GS (1989). Suicide in New York City nursing homes 1980-1986. *American Journal of Psychiatry* 145: 1487.

Alexopoulos GS, Abrams RC, Young RC, and Shamoian CA (1988). Cornell scale for depression in dementia. *Biological Psychiatry* 23: 271-284.

American Psychiatric Association Practice Guideline (1993). Practice guideline for major depressive disorder in adults. *American Journal of Psychiatry* 150: April 4 Supplement.

American Psychiatric Association (1998). Joint statement of the American Psychiatric Association and the American Association for Geriatric Psychiatry on the impact of the Omnibus Reconciliation Act of 1987 (OBRA '87) on psychiatric services in nursing homes. Presented to the Institute of Medicine Committee on Improving Quality of Life in Long-Term Care, March 12-13, Washington, DC.

Avorn J (1998). Depression in the elderly—falls and pitfalls (Editorial). *New England Journal of Medicine* 339: 918-920.

Borson S (1989). Reply to Abrams et al. *American Journal of Psychiatry* 145: 1487-1488.

Burke WJ, Roccaforte WH, Wengel SP, McArthur-Miller D, Folks DG, and Potter JE (1998). Disagreement in the reporting of depressive symptoms between patients with dementia of the Alzheimer type and their collateral sources. *American Journal of Geriatric Psychiatry* 6: 308-319.

Burns BJ and Kamerow DB (1988). Psychotropic drug prescriptions for nursing home residents. *Journal of Family Practice* 26: 155-160.

Carrol BJ (1998). The use of antidepressants in long-term care and the geriatric patient. *Geriatrics* 53: Supplement 4, S4-S11.

Conwell Y, Lyness JM, Duberstein P, Cox C, Seidlitz L, DiGiorgio A, and Caine ED (2000). Completed suicide among older patients in primary care practice. *Journal of the American Geriatrics Society* 48:23-29.

Costa e Silva J (1998). Randomized double-blind comparison of venlafaxine and fluoxetine in outpatients with major depression. *Journal of Clinical Psychiatry* 59: 352-357.

Haar A (1998). Health agency considers drug therapy guidelines (News report). *Provider* December: no volume, 14.

Habib A, Sanchez M, Pervez R, and Devanand DP (1998). Compliance with disposition to primary care physicians and psychiatrists in elderly homebound mentally ill patients. *American Journal of Geriatric Psychiatry* 6: 290-295.

Kettl PA (1999). Major depression: The forgotten illness. *Hospital Medicine* 35: 31-38.

Kidder SW and Kalachnik JE (1999). Regulation of inappropriate psychopharmacologic medication use in U.S. nursing homes from 1954 to 1997: Part II. *Annals of Long-Term Care* 7(2) 56-62.

Leipzig RM, Cummings RG, and Tinetti ME (1999). Drugs and falls in older people. *Journal of the American Geriatrics Society* 47: 30-39.

Loebel LP, Loebel JS, Dager SR, Centerwall BS, and Reay DT (1991). Anticipation of nursing home placement may be a precipitant of suicide among the elderly. *Journal of the American Geriatrics Society* 39: 407-408.

Lundquist G (1945). Prognosis and course in the manic-depressive psychoses. *Acta Psychiatrica et Neurologica Scandinavica* supplement 35: 1-96.

Medical Letter (1998). Citalopram for depression. *Medical Letter* 40: 113-114.

Murphy E (1983). The prognosis of depression in old age 1983. *British Journal of Psychiatry* 142: 111-119.

Parmalee PA, Katz IR, and Lawton MP (1989). Depression among institutionalized aged. *Journal of Gerontology* 1: M22-9.

Power CA and McCarron LT (1975). Treatment of depression in persons residing in homes for the aged. *Gerontologist* 15: 132-135.

Reynolds CF (1994). Treatment of depression in late life. *American Journal of Medicine 97* supplement 6A: 39S-46S.

Reynolds CF, Frank E, Dew MA, Houck PR, Miller M, Mazumdar S, Perel JM, and Kupfer DJ (1999). Treatment of 70+-year olds with recurrent major depression: Excellent short-term but brittle long-term response. *American Journal of Geriatric Psychiatry* 7: 64-69.

Roose SP, Laghrissi-Thode F, Kennedy JS, Nelson JC, Bigger JT, Pollock BG, Gaffney A, Narayen M, Finkel MS, McCafferty J, and Gergel I (1998). Comparison of paroxetine and nortriptyline in depressed patients with ischemic heart disease. *JAMA* 279: 287-291.

Thapa PB, Gideon P, Cost TW, Milam AB, and Ray WA (1998). Antidepressants and the risk of falls among nursing home residents. *New England Journal of Medicine* 339: 875-882.

Thompson LW, Gallagher D, Nies G, and Epstein D (1983). Evaluation of the effectiveness of professionals and non-professionals as instructors of coping with depression classes for elders. *Gerontologist* 23: 390-396.

Trappler B and Cohen CI (1998). Use of SSRI's in "very old" depressed nursing home residents. *American Journal of Geriatric Psychiatry* 6: 83-89.

Uncopher H, Levy ML, Skoloda T, Osgood NJ, Gallagher-Thompson D, and Bongar B (1998). Suicidal thoughts in male nursing home residents. *Annals of Long-Term Care* 6: 301-308.

Yesavage JA, Brink TL, Rose TL, Lum O, Huang V, Adey M, and Leirer VD (1983). Development and validation of a geriatric screening tool. *Journal of Psychiatry*.

Chapter 14

Bundlie SR (1998). Sleep in aging. *Geriatrics 53* supplement 11: 541-543.

Cohen D, Eisdorfer C, Prinz P, Breen A, Davis M, and Gadsby A (1983). Sleep disturbances in the institutionalized aged. *Journal of the American Geriatrics Society* 31: 79-82.

Cohen G (1998). Anxiety in Alzheimer's disease (Editorial). *American Journal of Geriatric Psychiatry* 6: 1-4.

Cruise PA, Schnelle JF, Alessi C, Simmons SF, and Ouslander JG (1999). The nighttime environment and incontinence care practices in nursing homes. *Journal of the American Geriatrics Society* 46: 181-186.

Folks DG (1999a). Management of insomnia in the long-term care setting. *Annals of Long-Term Care* 7: 7-13.

Folks DG (1999b). Management of anxiety in the long-term care setting. *Annals of Long-Term Care* 7: 439-441.

Forsell Y and Winblad B (1997). Anxiety disorders in demented and non-demented elderly patients: Prevalence and correlates (Letter). *Journal of Neurology, Neurosurgery and Psychiatry* 62: 294-295.

Luchins DJ and Rose RP (1989). Late-life onset of panic disorder with agoraphobia in three patients. *American Journal of Psychiatry* 146: 920-921.

Opedal K, Schjøtt J, and Eide E (1998). Use of hypnotics among patients in geriatric institutions. *International Journal of Geriatric Psychiatry* 13: 846-851.

Regenstein QR and Morris J (1987). Daily sleep patterns observed among institutionalized elderly residents. *Journal of the American Geriatrics Society* 35: 767-772.

Sadavoy J and Dorion B (1984). Treatment of the elderly characterologically disturbed patient in the chronic care institution. *Journal of Geriatric Psychiatry* 16: 223-240.

Waldhorn R (1989). Incidence of sleep disorders in nursing home patients (News item). *Geriatric Consultant* 8: 6-7.

Wands K, Merskey HA, Hachinski VC, Fisman M, Fox H, and Bonifero M (1990). A questionnaire investigation of anxiety and depression in early dementia. *Journal of the American Geriatrics Society* 47: 131-138.

Chapter 15

Braun JA (1999). Legal aspects of restraint use in nursing homes. *Untie the Elderly* 11 1-3. Full citations from <jabraun@ameritech.net>.

Brody EM, Kleban MH, and Moss MS (1984). Predictors of falls among institutionalized women with Alzheimer's disease. *Journal of the American Geriatrics Society* 32: 877-882.

Caramel VMB, Remarque EJ, Knook DL, Lagaay AM, and Van den Brande KJ (1998). Benzodiazepine users aged 85 and older fall more often (Letter). *Journal of the American Geriatrics Society* 46: 1178-1179.

Evans LK and Strumpf NE (1989). Tying down the elderly. *Journal of the American Geriatrics Society* 37: 65-74.

Frengley JD and Mion LC (1986). Incidence of physical restraints on acute general medical wards. *Journal of the American Geriatrics Society* 34: 565-569.

Gold S, Gordon B, and Silber M (1988). If a patient falls from her wheelchair, is expert medical evidence needed to establish nursing home's negligence? *Physician's Medical Law Letter,* New York: Professional Liability Publications Co. January issue: 1-4.

Granek E, Baker SP, Abbey H, Robinson E, Myers AH, Samkoff JS, and Klein LE (1987). Medications and diagnoses in relation to falls in a long-term care facility. *Journal of the American Geriatrics Society* 35: 503-511.

Grossberg GT (1993). The impact of OBRA on the use of physical restraints (Editorial). *Nursing Home Medicine* 1: 1.

Hesse KA and Campion EW (1983). Motivating the geriatric patient for rehabilitation. *Journal of the American Geriatrics Society* 31: 586-589.

Kapp MB (1999). Restraint reduction and legal risk management. *Journal of the American Geriatrics Society* 47: 375-376.

Klein DE, Steinberg M, Galik E, Steele C, Sheppard JM, Warren A, Rosenblatt A, and Lyketsos CG (1999). Wandering behavior in community-residing persons with dementia. *International Journal of Geriatric Psychiatry* 14: 272-279.

Leipzig RM, Cummings RG, and Tinetti ME (1999). Drugs and falls in older people. *Journal of the American Geriatrics Society* 47: 30-39.

Lyon LL and Nevins MA (1984). Management of hip fractures in nursing home patients. *Journal of the American Geriatrics Society* 32: 391-395.

Miles S and Parker K (1998). Deaths caused by bed rails: Reply to Plichta (Letter). *Journal of the American Geriatrics Society* 46: 794.

Nickens HW (1983). A review of factors affecting the occurrence and outcome of hip fracture with special reference to psychosocial issues. *Journal of the American Geriatrics Society* 31: 166-170.

Pawlson LG, Goodwin M, and Keith K (1986). Wheelchair use by ambulatory nursing home residents. *Journal of the American Geriatrics Society* 34: 860-864.

Plichta AM (1998). Deaths caused by bed rails (Letter). *Journal of the American Geriatrics Society* 46: 794.

Robbins AS, Rubenstein LZ, Josephson KR, Schulman BL, Osterweil D, and Fine G (1989). Predictors of falls among elderly people. *Archives of Internal Medicine* 149: 1628-1633.

Rudman IW and Rudman D (1989). High rate of fractures for men in nursing homes. *American Journal of Physical Medicine and Rehabilitation* 68: 2-5.

Schnelle JF, Simmons SF, and Ory MG (1992). Risk factors that predict staff failure to release nursing home residents from restraints. *Gerontologist* 32: 767-770.

Selikson S, Damus K, and Hammerman D (1988). Risk factors associated with immobility. *Journal of the American Geriatrics Society* 36: 707-712.

Sullivan-Marx EM, Strumpf NE, Evans LK, Baumgarten M, and Maislin G (1999). Predictors of continued physical restraint use in nursing home residents following restraint reduction efforts. *Journal of the American Geriatrics Society* 47: 342-348.

Tammalleo AD (1988). Patient wanders off: Killed by daughter. *Fields v. Senior Citizens Center Inc.* Regan Reports on Nursing Law: 29: 2.

Thapa PB, Gideon P, Cost TW, Milam AB, and Ray WA (1998). Antidepressants and the risk of falls among nursing home residents. *New England Journal of Medicine* 339: 875-882.

Tideiksaar R (1986). Nursing home falls and investigation of the single and multiple faller (Abstract). *Journal of the American Geriatrics Society* 34: 675.

Tideiksaar R (1998). *Falls in older persons: Prevention and management.* Baltimore: Health Profession Press.

Tideiksaar R and Osterwell D (1989). Prevention of bed falls. *Geriatric Medicine Today* 8: 70-78.

Tinetti ME (1987). Factors associated with serious injury during falls by ambulatory nursing home residents. *Journal of the American Geriatrics Society* 35: 644-648.

Tinetti ME, Speechley M, and Ginter NF (1988). Risk factors for falls among elderly persons living in the community. *New England Journal of Medicine* 26: 1701-1707.

Tinetti ME and Williams CS (1997). Falls, injuries due to falls, and the risk of admission to a nursing home. *New England Journal of Medicine* 337: 1279-1284.

Chapter 16

Billig W, Cohen-Mansfield J, and Lipson S (1991). Pharmacological treatment of agitation in a nursing home. *Journal of the American Geriatrics Society* 39: 1002-1005.

Burke WH and Lewis FD (1986). Management of maladaptive social behavior of a brain-injured adult. *International Journal of Rehabilitation Research* 9: 335-342.

Burke WH and Wesolowski MD (1988). Applied behavior analysis in head injury rehabilitation. *Rehabilitation Nursing* 13: 186-188.

Burns A, Jacoby R, and Levy R (1990). Psychiatric phenomena in Alzheimer's disease. *British Journal of Psychiatry* 157: 86-94.

Butterfield F (1997). America's aging violent prisoners. *The New York Times,* July 6.

Butterfield F (1998). Prisons replace hospitals for the nation's mentally ill. *The New York Times,* March 5.

Gardner ME, Ditmanson L, and Baker A (1998). Effectiveness of divalproex sodium in the treatment of aggressive behaviors in dementia. Poster exhibit, American Medical Directors Association Annual Meeting, Tucson, AZ.

Garner ME and Garrett RW (1997). Review of drug therapy for aggressive behaviors associated with dementia. *Nursing Home Medicine* 5 199-207.

Goldstein K (1952). The effect of brain damage on the personality. *Psychiatry* 15: 245-260.

Gormley N, Rizwan MR, and Lovestone S (1998). Clinical predictors of aggressive behavior in Alzheimer's disease. *International Journal of Geriatric Psychiatry* 12: 109-115.

Green RG and Kellerman AL (1996). Grandfather's gun: When should we intervene. *Journal of the American Geriatrics Society* 44: 467-469.

Greenwald BS, Marin D, and Silverman S (1986). Serotoninergic treatment of screaming and banging in dementia. *Lancet* 2(8521-22): 1464-1465.

Habib A, Birkett DP, and Devanand D (1998). Late onset mania. *Clinical Gerontologist* 16: 43-48.

Hanger HC and Mulley GP (1993). Questions people ask about stroke. *Stroke* 24: 536-538.

Herrmann N and Eryavec G (1993). Buspirone in the management of agitation and aggression associated with dementia. *American Journal of Geriatric Psychiatry* 1: 249-253.

Houlihan DJ, Mulsant BH, Sweet RA, Rifai AH, Pasternak R, Rosen J, and Zubenko, GS (1994). A naturalistic study of trazodone in the treatment of behavioral complications of dementia. *American Journal of Geriatric Psychiatry* 2: 78-85.

Isaac RJ and Armat VC (1990). *Madness in the streets.* New York: Free Press.

Isaacs B, Neville Y, and Rushford I (1976). The stricken: The social consequences of stroke. *Age and Ageing* 5: 188-192.

Lawlor B (1998). The use of selective serotonin reuptake inhibitors for depression and psychosis complicating dementia (Letter). *International Journal of Geriatric Psychiatry* 13: 496.

Lyketsos CG, Steele C, Galik E, Rosenblatt A, Steinberg M, Warren A, and Sheppard JM (1999). Physical aggression in dementia patients and its relationship to depression. *American Journal of Psychiatry* 156: 66-71.

Marin DB and Greenwald DS (1989). Carbamezapine for aggressive agitation in demented patients during nursing care. *American Journal of Psychiatry* 146: 805.

McElroy S, Kasckow JW, Lott AD, and Keck PE (1996). Valproate in the treatment of behavioral agitation of dementia. *Psychiatric Annals* 26: S474-S478.

Mesnikoff A and Wilder D (1983). "Behavior problems encountered in adult homes." In Aronson MK, Bennett R, and Gurland B (Eds.), (pp. 29-37). *The acting-out elderly.* Binghamton, NY: The Haworth Press.

Mintzer JE, Hoernig KS, and Mirski DF (1998). Treatment of agitation in patients with dementia. *Clinics in Geriatric Medicine* 14: 147-175.

Nilsson K, Palmstierna T, and Wisted B (1988). Aggressive behavior in hospitalized psychogeriatric patients. *Acta Psychiatrica Scandinavica* 78: 172-175.

Patel V and Hope RA (1992). A rating scale for aggressive behavior in the elderly—the RAGE. *Psychological Medicine* 22: 211-221.

Patterson JF (1987). Carbamezapine for assaultive patients with organic brain disease: An open pilot study. *Psychosomatics* 28: 579-581.

Petrie WM, Lawson EC, and Hollender MH (1982). Violence in geriatric patients. *JAMA* 248: 443-444.

Pinner E and Rich CI (1988). Effects of trazodone on aggressive behavior in seven patients with organic mental disorder. *American Journal of Psychiatry* 145: 1295-1296.

Porsteinsson AP, Tariot PN, Erb R, and Gaile S (1997). An open trial of valproate for agitation in geriatric neuropsychiatric disorders. *American Journal of Geriatric Psychiatry* 5: 344-351.

Ryden MB (1988). Aggressive behavior in persons with dementia who live in the community. *Alzheimer Disease and Related Disorders* 2: 342-355.

Schneider L, Pollock VE, and Lyness SA (1990). A metaanalysis of controlled trials of neuroleptic treatment in dementia. *Journal of the American Geriatrics Society* 38: 555-563.

Shah AK (1993). Aggressive behavior among patients referred to a psychogeriatric service. *Medicine, Science and the Law* 33, 144-150.

Sharma N, Rosman H, Padhi D, and Tisdale J (1998). Torsade de pointes associated with intravenous haloperidol in critically ill patients. *American Journal of Cardiology* 81: 238-240.

Thacker S (1996). Junior doctors and emergency tranquillisation of elderly confused patients: A survey. *Psychiatric Bulletin* 20: 212-214.

Thomas H, Schwartz E, and Petrilli R (1992). Droperidol versus haloperidol for chemical restraint of agitated and combative patients. *Annals of Emergency Medicine* 21: 407-413.

Tsai S-J, Hwang J-P, Yang C-H, and Liu K-M (1996). Physical aggression and associated factors in probable Alzheimer disease. *Alzheimer Disease and Associated Disorders* 10: 82-85.

Yudofsky S, Williams D, and Gorman J (1981). Propranolol in the treatment of rage and violent behavior in patients with chronic brain syndrome. *American Journal of Psychiatry* 138: 218-220.

Yudovsky SC, Silver JM, and Hales RE (1990). Pharmacological management of aggression in the elderly. *Journal of Clinical Psychiatry* 51 supplement: 22-28.

Chapter 17

Agronin ME and Maletta G (2000). Personality disorders in late life. *American Journal of Geriatric Psychiatry* 8: 4-18.

Alessi CA and Henderson CT (1988). Constipation and fecal impaction in the long-term care patient. *Clinics in Geriatric Medicine* 4: 571-588.

Alexopoulos GS, Silver JM, Kahn DA, et al eds (1998). Treatment of agitation in older persons with dementia. The expert consensus guidelines series. *Postgraduate Medicine:* Special report.

Bliwise DL, Carroll JS, Lee KA, Nekich JC, and Dement WC (1993). Sleep and "sundowning" in nursing home patients with dementia. *Psychiatry Research* 48: 277-292.

Burgio L, Scilley C, Hardin JM, Hsu C, and Yancey J (1996). Environmental "white noise": An intervention for verbally agitated nursing home residents. *Journal of Gerontology—Psychological Sciences* 51B: 364-373.

Cameron O (1941). Studies in senile nocturnal delirium. *Psychiatric Quarterly* 15: 47-53.

Christensen DB and Benfield WR (1998). Alprazolam as an alernative to low-dose haloperidol in older cognitively impaired nursing facility residents. *Journal of the American Geriatrics Society* 46: 620-625.

Cohen-Mansfield J (1986). Agitated behaviors in the elderly II. *Journal of the American Geriatrics Society* 34: 722-727.

Cohen-Mansfield J, Marx MS, and Rosenthal AS (1989). A description of agitation in a nursing home. *Journal of Gerontology* 44: M77-84.

Cooper AJ (1987). Medroxyprogesterone acetate treatment of sexual acting out in men suffering from dementia. *Journal of Clinical Psychiatry* 48: 368-370.

Cruise PA, Schnelle JF, Alessi C, Simmons SF, and Ouslander JG (1998). The nighttime environment and incontinence care practices in nursing homes. *Journal of the American Geriatrics Society* 46: 181-186.

Evans LK (1987). Sundown syndrome in the institutionalized elderly. *Journal of the American Geriatrics Society* 35: 101-108.

Fatis M, Smasai MS, and Betts BJ (1989). Behavioral psychological intervention. *Journal of Gerontological Nursing* 15: 25-28.

Gibb WRG (1989). Dementia and Parkinson's disease. *British Journal of Psychiatry* 154: 596-614.

Goldberg RL (1999). The use of adjunctive divalproex for neuroleptic unresponsive behavioral disturbances in nursing home residents with dementia. *Annals of Long-Term Care* 7: 63-66.

Harwood DG, Ownby RL, Barker WW, and Duara R (1998). The behavioral pathology in Alzheimer's disease scale (Behave-AD): Factor structure among community-dwelling Alzheimer's disease patients. *International Journal of Geriatric Psychiatry* 13: 793-800.

Herrmann N (1998). Not just neuroleptics: The use of antiepileptics in dementia. *Old Age Psychiatrist* 13: 6.

Hope T, Keene J, Fairburn CG, Jacoby R, and McShane R (1999). Natural history of behavioral changes and psychiatric symptoms in Alzheimer's disease. *British Journal of Psychiatry* 174: 39-44.

Hwang J-P, Trai S-J, Yang C-H, Liu K-M, and Lirng J-F (1998). Hoarding behavior in dementia. *American Journal of Geriatric Psychiatry* 6: 285-289.

Jensen CE (1989). Sexual agitation in Alzheimer's disease. *Journal of the American Geriatrics Society* 37: 917-918

Kane RA, Wilson KB, and Clemmer E (1993). Assisted Living in the United States: A New Paradigm for Residential Care for Frail Older Persons? Report by Public Policy Institute, American Association of Retired Persons.

Katz IR, Sands LP, Bilker W, Di Filippo S, Boyce A, and D'Angelo K (1998). Identification of medicines that cause cognitive impairment in older people: The case of oxybutynin chloride. *Journal of the American Geriatrics Society* 46: 8-13.

Kyomen HH, Nobel KW, and Wei JY (1991). The use of estrogen to decrease aggressive physical behavior in elderly men with dementia. *Journal of the American Geriatrics Society* 39: 1110-1112.

Lackner T, Roach MB, and Kennedy KL (2000). Managing urinary incontinence in the geriatric patient with overactive bladder. *Nursing Home Medicine* unpaged supplement to January issue. Plainsboro, NJ: MultiMedia HealthCare/Freedom LLC.

Levitsky AM and Owens NJ (1999). Pharmacologic treatment of hypersexuality and paraphilias in nursing home residents. *Journal of the American Geriatrics Society* 47: 231-234.

Lund and Manchester Groups, no authors listed (1994). Clinical and neuropathological criteria for frontotemporal dementia. *Journal of Neurology, Neurosurgery, and Psychiatry* 57: 416-418.

McCartney JR (1999). Hoarding requires special attention. *Brown University GeroPsych Report* 3(7): 1-6.

Molinari V, Kunik ME, Mulsant B, and Rifai AH (1998). The relationship between patient, informant, social worker and consensus diagnosis of personality disorder in elderly depressed inpatients. *American Journal of Geriatric Psychiatry* 6: 136-144.

Morley JE (1999). Update on nursing home care. *Annals of Long-Term Care* 7: 16-19.

National Institutes of Health (1988). "Urinary incontinence in adults." National Institutes of Health Consensus Development Conference Statement. Volume 7, Number 5, October.

Nilsson K, Palmstierna T, and Wisted B (1988). Aggressive behavior in hospitalized psychogeriatric patients. *Acta Psychiatrica Scandinavica* 78: 172-175.

Raji M, Liu D, and Wallace D (2000). Sexual aggressiveness in a patient with dementia. *Annals of Long-Term Care* 8: 81-83.

Ribeiro DJ and Smith SR (1985). Evaluation of urinary catheterization and urinary incontinence in a general nursing home population. *Journal of the American Geriatrics Society* 33: 479-488.

Rohrer JE, Buckwalter K, and Russell D (1989). The effects of mental dysfunction on nursing home care. *Social Science and Medicine* 28: 399-403.

Rosen J, Burgio L, Kollar M, Cain M, Allison M, Fogleman M, Michael M, and Zubenko GS (1994). The Pittsburgh Agitation Scale. *American Journal of Geriatric Psychiatry* 2: 52-59.

Ryan DP, Tainsh SM, Kolodny V, and Lendrum BL (1988). Noise-making amongst the elderly in long-term care. *Gerontologist* 3: 369-371.

Sloane PD, Davidson S, Knight N, Tangen C, and Mitchell CM (1999). Severe disruptive vocalizers. *Journal of the American Geriatrics Society* 47: 439-445.

Smith RG (1983). Fecal incontinence. *Journal of the American Geriatrics Society* 31: 694-697.

Steinke EE (1997). Sexuality in aging: Implications for nursing facility staff. *Journal of Continuing Education in Nursing* 28: 59-63.

Stewart JT and Shin KJ (1997). Paroxetine treatment of sexual disinhibition in dementia (Letter). *American Journal of Psychiatry* 154: 1474.

Swearer JM, Drachman DA, O'Donnell BF, and Mitchell AL (1988). Troublesome and disruptive behaviors in dementia relationships to diagnosis and disease severity. *Journal of the American Geriatrics Society* 36: 784-790.

Szasz G (1983). Sexual incidents in an extended care unit for aged men. *Journal of the American Geriatrics Society* 31: 407-411.

Warren JW, Muncie HL, and Hall-Craggs M (1988). Acute pyelonephritis associated with the bacteruria of long-term catheterization. *Journal of Infectious Disease* 158: 1341-1346.

Wasow M and Loeb MB (1979). Sexuality in nursing homes. *Journal of the American Geriatrics Society* 27: 73-79.

Werner P, Hay DP, and Cohen-Mansfield J (1995). Management of disruptive vocalizations in the nursing home. *Nursing Home Medicine* 3: 217-225.

Work Group on Alzheimer's Disease and Related Dementias (1997). Practice guidelines for the treatment of Alzheimer's disease and other dementias of late life. *American Journal of Psychiatry* Supplement: 154.

Zimmer JA, Watson N, and Treat A (1984). Behavioral problems among patients in skilled nursing facilities. *American Journal of Public Health* 74: 1118-1121.

Chapter 18

American Medical Directors Association (1999). Chronic Pain Management Clinical Practice Guideline. <www.amda.com>.

Benjamin AE (1988). Long-term care and AIDS perspectives from experience with the elderly. *Milbank Quarterly* 66: 415-443.

Bennett RG, O'Sullivan J, Devito E, and Remsberg R (2000). The increasing medical malpractice risk related to pressure ulcers in the United States. *Journal of the American Geriatrics Society* 48: 73-81.

Bernabei R, Gambassi G, Lapane K, Landi F, Gatsonis C, Dunlop R, Lipsitz L, Steel K, and Mor V (1998). Management of pain in elderly patients with cancer. *JAMA* 279: 1877-1882.

Campbell-Taylor I and Fisher HR (1988). The clinical case against tube feeding in palliative care of the elderly. *Journal of the American Geriatrics Society* 35: 1100-1103.

Cogen RE (1988). Tube feeding in patients with advanced and terminal neurological disease (Letter). *Journal of the American Geriatrics Society* 36: 574.

Endres J, Poon SW, and Welch P (1989). Diabetics in long-term care: Effect of sweetness on dietary intake. *Annals of the New York Academy of Science* 561: 157-161.

Engle VF, Fox-Hill E, and Graney MJ (1998). The experience of living-dying in a nursing home: Self-reports of black and white older adults. *Journal of the American Geriatrics Society* 46: 1091-1096.

Ferrell BA (1998). Pressure ulcer products and devices: Are they safe, much less effective? *Journal of the American Geriatrics Society* 46: 654-655.

Fisman DN, Levy AR, Gifford DR, and Tamblyn R (1999). Survival after percutaneous endoscopic gastrostomy among older residents of Quebec. *Journal of the American Geriatrics Society* 47: 349-353.

Franklin CA and Karbeck J (1989). Weight loss and senile dementia in an institutionalized elderly population. *Journal of the American Dietetic Association* 89: 790-792.

Gillick MR (2000). Rethinking the role of tube feeding in patients with advanced dementia. *New England Journal of Medicine* 342: 206-210.

Marion Merrill Dow Managed Care Digest. Long-Term Care Edition (1991). Kansas City, MO: Marion Merrill Dow.

Mason K (1991). Identifying and providing for today's long-term care resident. *Provider* August, no volume 25-37.

Morley JE (1999). Update on nursing home care. *Annals of Long-Term Care* 7: 16-19.

Morris CH, Hope RA, and Fairburn CG (1989). Eating habits in dementia. *British Journal of Psychiatry* 154: 801-806.

Nash D, Broome J, and Stone S (1987). Behavior modification of pica in a geriatric patient. *Journal of the American Geriatrics Society* 35: 79-80.

New York State Department of Health (1988). *A physician's guide to AIDS: Issues in the medical office.*

Norberg A, Backstrom A, Athlin E, and Norberg B (1988). Food refusal amongst nursing home patients as conceptualized by nurses aides and enrolled nurses. *Journal of Advanced Nursing* 13: 478-483.

Rozzini R, Bianchetti A, Zanetti O, and Trabucchi M (1989). Are too many drugs prescribed for the elderly after all? *Journal of the American Geriatrics Society* 37: 89-90.

Spagnoli A, Ostino G, Borga AD, D'Ambrosio R, Maggiorotti P, Todisco E, Prattichizzo W, Pia L, and Comelli M (1989). Drug compliance and unreported drugs in the elderly. *Journal of the American Geriatrics Society* 37: 619-624.

Thomas DR, Kamel H, and Morley JE (1998). Nutritional deficiencies in long-term care: Part III. *Annals of Long-Term Care* 6 (supplement): S1-S8.

Chapter 19

Birkett DP (1996). *The Psychiatry of Stroke.* Washington, DC: American Psychiatric Press.

Lackner TE, Cloyd JC, Thomas LW, and Leppik IE (1998). Antiepileptic drug use in nursing home residents: Effects of age, gender and co-medication on patterns of use. *Epilepsia* 39 (10): 1083-1087.

Lasser RA and Sunderland T (1998). Newer psychotropic medication use in nursing home residents. *Journal of the American Geriatrics Society* 46: 202-207.

Rizzolo PJ and Snow T (1989). Use of a hearing assistance device in nursing homes. *American Family Physician* 39: 227-229.

Robey RR (1998). A meta-analysis of clinical outcomes in the treatment of aphasia. *Journal of Speech Language and Hearing Research* 41: 172-187.

Chapter 20

Agüero-Torres H, Fratiglioni L, and Winblad B (1998). Natural history of Alzheimer's disease and other dementias. *International Journal of Geriatric Psychiatry* 13: 755-766.

Barry PB, Crescenzi CA, Radovsky L, Kern DC, and Stee K (1988). Why elderly patients refuse hospitalization. *Journal of the American Geriatrics Society* 36: 419-424.

Bowker L, Stewart K, Hayes S, and Gill M (1998). Do general practitioners know when living wills are legal? *Journal of the Royal College of Physicians of London* 32: 492-493.

Bradley EH, Peiris V, and Wetle T (1998). Discussions about end-of-life care in nursing homes. *Journal of the American Geriatrics Society* 46: 1235-1241.

Downe-Wamboldt B, Butler L, and Coughlan S (1998). Nurses' knowledge, experiences, and attitudes concerning living wills. *Canadian Journal of Nursing Research* 30: 161-175.

Engle VF, Fox-Hill E, and Graney MJ (1998). The experience of living-dying in a nursing home: Self-reports of black and white older adults. *Journal of the American Geriatrics Society* 46: 1091-1096.

Fader MF, Gambert SR, Nash M, Gupta KL, and Escher J (1989). Implementing a DNR policy in a nursing home. *Journal of the American Geriatrics Society* 37: 544-548.

Finne-Soveri UH and Tilvis RS (1998). How accurate is the terminal prognosis in the minimum data set? *Journal of the American Geriatrics Society* 46: 1023-1024.

Finucane TE and Denman SJ (1989). Deciding to abort resuscitation in a nursing home. *Journal of the American Geriatrics Society* 37: 684-688.

Fried TR, Pollack DM, Drickamer MA, and Tinetti ME (1999). Who dies at home? Determinants of site of death for community-based long-term care patients. *Journal of the American Geriatrics Society* 47: 25-29.

Fried TR, Van Doorn C, O'Leary JR, Tinetti ME, and Drickamer MA (1999). Older persons' perceptions of home and hospital as sites of treatment for acute illness. *American Journal of Medicine* 107: 317-323.

Gabow PA, Hutt DM, Baker S, Craig SR, Gordon JR, and Lezotte DC (1985). Comparison of hospitalization between nursing home and community residents. *Journal of the American Geriatrics Society* 33: 524-530.

Gillick M, Berkman S, and Cullen R (1999). A patient-centered approach to advance medical planning in the nursing home. *Journal of the American Geriatrics Society* 47: 227-230.

Gillick MR, Serell NA, and Gillick LS (1982). Adverse consequences of hospitalization in the elderly. *Social Science and Medicine* 16: 1033-1038.

Himber CP (1989). The right to die needs protection. *The New York Times* (New Jersey Section), January 9.

Horowitz AC (1992). New law obligates providers to inform residents of rights. *Provider* 18: 36.

Katz PR (1989). The real meaning of home in nursing home. *Journal of the American Geriatrics Society* 37: 665.

Levenson SA and Feinsod FM (1998). Obtaining instructions for care. *Annals of Long-Term Care* 6: 295-300.

Levin JR, Wenger NS, Ouslander JG, Zellman G, Schnelle C, Buchanan JL, Hirsch SH, and Reuben DB (1999). Life-sustaining treatment decisions for nursing home residents. *Journal of the American Geriatrics Society* 47: 82-87.

Ouslander JG, Tymchuk AJ, and Rahbar H (1989). Health care decisions among elderly longterm care residents and their proxies. *Archives of Internal Medicine* 149: 1367-1372.

Ouslander JG, Weinberg AD, and Philips V (2000). Inappropriate hospitalization of nursing facility residents (Editorial). *Journal of the American Geriatrics Society* 48: 230-231.

Pritchard RS, Fisher SE, Teno JM, Sharp SM, Reding DJ, Knaus WA, Wennberg JE, and Lynn J (1998). Influence of patient preferences and local health system characteristics on the place of death. *Journal of the American Geriatrics Society* 46: 1242-1250.

Reuben DB, Schnelle JF, Buchanan JL, Kington RS, Zellman GI, Farley DO, Hirsch SH, and Ouslander JG (1999). Primary care of long-stay nursing home residents. *Journal of the American Geriatrics Society* 47: 131-138.

Rodgman E (1996). The use of living wills at the end of life. A national study. *Archives of Internal Medicine* 156: 1018-1022.

Sansone P, Schmitt L, Nichols J, Philips M, and Belisle S (1998). Determining the capacity of demented nursing home residents to name a health care proxy. *Clinical Gerontologist* 19(4): 35-50.

Shields T (1995). Dutch hospitals face up to living wills (news). *BMJ* 310: 82.

Sickbert S (1989). Coronary care visitation and summary of the literature. *Journal of the American Geriatrics Society* 37: 655-657.

Teno JM (1998). Looking beyond the form to complex interventions needed to improve end of life care (Editorial). *Journal of the American Geriatrics Society* 46: 1170-1171.

Tresch DD, Simpson WM, and Burton JR (1985). Relationship of long-term and acute care facilities. *Journal of the American Geriatrics Society* 33: 819-827.

VandeCreek L, Frankowski D, and Johnson M (1995). Variables that predict interest in and completion of living wills. *Journal of Pastoral Care* 49: 212-220.

Wolff ML, Smolen S, and Ferrara L (1985). Treatment decisions in a skilled nursing facility. *Journal of the American Geriatrics Society* 33: 440-445.

Chapter 21

Anderson DS (1999). Dementia care in the UK—a single service for all. *International Journal of Geriatric Psychiatry* 14: 1-2.

Cassel CK (1985). Research in nursing homes. *Journal of the American Geriatrics Society* 33: 795-799.

Hasle H and Olsen RB (1989). Consumption of psychopharmacologicals by residents at nursing homes. *Ugeskrift for Laeger* 151: 1313-1316.

Hepple J, Bowler I, and Bowman CE (1989). A survey of private nursing home residents in Weston Super Mare. *Age and Ageing* 18: 61-63.

Hodkinson E, McCafferty SG, Scott JN, and Stout RW (1988). Disability and dependency in elderly people in residential and hospital care. *Age and Ageing* 17:147-154.

Jolley DJ (1999). Care of older people with mental illness. *Psychiatric Bulletin* 23: 117-120.

Karlawish JHT, Hougham GW, Stocking CB, and Sachs GA (1999). What is the quality of reporting of research ethics in publications of nursing home research? *Journal of the American Geriatrics Society* 47: 76-81.

Lau-Ting C, Ting T, and Phoon WO (1987). Mental status of residents in old people's homes. *Annals of the Academy of Medicine of Singapore* 16: 118-121.

Lehmkuhl D, Bosch G, and Steinhart I (1986). Old people in homes. *Zeitschrift Gerontologie* 19: 56-64.

Libow LS (1984). The teaching nursing home past present and future. *Journal of the American Geriatrics Society.* 32: 598-603.

Nolan L and O'Malley K (1989). The need for a more rational approach to drug prescribing for elderly people in nursing homes. *Age and Ageing* 18: 52-56.

Perkins RE, King SA, and Hollyman JA (1989). Resettlement of long-stay psychiatric patients the use of the private sector. *British Journal of Psychiatry* 155: 233-238.

Rabins PV, Rovner BW, Larson DB, Burns BJ, Prescott C, and Bearsley RS (1987). The use of mental health measures in nursing home research. *Journal of the American Geriatrics Society* 35: 431-434.

Wagner L (2000). Meeting the baby boomer challenge. *Provider* 26: 29-38.

Wayne SJ, Rhyne RI, Thompson RE, and Davis M (1991). Sampling issues in nursing home reasearch. *Journal of the American Geriatrics Society* 39: 308-311.

Index

Page numbers followed by the letter "t" indicate tables.

Printed in the United States
by Baker & Taylor Publisher Services

Printed in the United States
by Baker & Taylor Publisher Services